Exclusively Pumping Breast Milk

A Guide to Providing Expressed Breast Milk for Your Baby

Second Edition

Exclusively Pumping Breast Milk

A Guide to Providing Expressed Breast Milk for Your Baby

Second Edition

Stephanie Casemore

GRAY LION PUBLISHING
Napanee, Ontario, Canada

Published by Gray Lion Publishing
Napanee, Ontario, Canada
www.exclusivelypumping.com

Some material in this book has been adapted from material previously published in *Breastfeeding, Take Two: Successful Breastfeeding the Second Time Around* copyright © Stephanie Casemore 2012, specifically Chapter 3: The Emotions of Exclusively Pumping and Chapter 4: Lactation and Breast Milk Composition

Library and Archives Canada Cataloguing in Publication
Casemore, Stephanie, 1971-, author
    Exclusively pumping breast milk: a guide to providing expressed breast milk for your baby / Stephanie Casemore. -- Second edition.
Includes bibliographical references and index.
ISBN 978-0-9736142-2-0 (pbk.)
1. Breast milk--Collection and preservation. 2. Breast pumps. I. Title.
RJ216.C345 2014   649'.33   C2013-904199-0

Editing by Sharon Dewey Hetke
Cover design by Diane McIntosh, Bright Ideas

The information presented in this book is based on the personal experience of the author. If you require medical advice, or other expert assistance, you should seek the services of a competent professional. Before taking any course of action that may affect you, or your baby, it is strongly advised that you consult with a medical professional.

To all the strong, determined, committed, loving mothers who continually amaze, encourage, and inspire me.

— S.C.

Table of Contents

Introduction to the Second Edition

I t's hard to believe that almost ten years have passed since publishing the first edition of *Exclusively Pumping Breast Milk*. Over those years, many things have changed and many have stayed the same.

The option of exclusively pumping as an alternative to formula feeding has made small but steady gains in terms of recognition and acceptance, yet at the same time many women are still unaware of this opportunity to provide breast milk for their babies when breastfeeding doesn't work out or isn't desired. I still receive far too many emails in which women lament that they thought they were the only ones exclusively expressing breast milk for their little ones. My earnest hope is that exclusively pumping will become accepted in the medical and lactation communities for what it is—an alternative to formula feeding—and that expectant mothers will be informed of the option during prenatal and breastfeeding classes. Far too often it is seen as competing with breastfeeding, and while some women will choose to exclusively pump instead of breastfeed, the vast majority of exclusively pumping mothers are women who wanted to breastfeed but were faced with challenges they had difficulty overcoming. When we have accurate information and meaningful breastfeeding support for every new mother, and a society that accepts and supports breastfeeding not just as a token but in meaningful ways, then fewer women will exclusively pump. But until then this is an option that needs to be supported and shared.

Sharing has become easier over the past ten years as the internet has grown and become the go-to source of information for many new moms. What would we do without it? As a tool, it is providing women the opportunity to research information about pumping and lactation, resulting in more well-informed mothers. However, the internet also leaves new mothers open and vulnerable to a plethora of inaccurate information, and so now, more than ever, it is necessary to find information that is from a reliable and trusted source—not always easy to do. As a communication device, the internet provides a valuable connection between women, offering support and camaraderie where it was once difficult to find. No longer do women need to go it alone. Regardless of your situation, you will find others who understand and have first-hand experience with what you are going through. You will find information and support online and do not ever need to feel isolated when exclusively pumping.

While there has been some research conducted over the past few years relating to expressing breast milk, most is, unfortunately, still not directly relating to long-term exclusive breast milk expression. Instead, research tends to be focused on the use of breast pumps to initiate milk production in moms of premature infants or is funded by pump companies attempting to prove the efficacy of their own pumps. Some of this information is still relevant to exclusively pumping mothers, but it is my hope that before the third edition of this book is released we will see an acknowledgement of the number of women who are exclusively pumping—and specific research on the topic. Having said that, this new edition does provide a significant increase in the number of sources cited, with endnotes provided for both sources and additional information.

On a personal note, the past ten years have brought a number of changes. My second child was born in 2006 and although I was worried that I might again experience breastfeeding difficulties, these fears proved unfounded. My daughter breastfed for just over three years, and while I had a lot to do in order to work through the emotional baggage I brought with me from my first experience exclusively pumping for my son, I also gained a great deal of wisdom from the experience. Most importantly, I began to clearly understand the emotional aspects of breastfeeding — and not breastfeeding — and to recognize how breastfeeding affects not only our children but also us as mothers. Noting a void in current breastfeeding literature, I set out to write a book on the topic and to support mothers who have had past breastfeeding challenges move into their next breastfeeding experience with a sense of empowerment and knowledge. *Breastfeeding, Take Two: Successful Breastfeeding the Second Time Around* is the result of my experience with my daughter, but was initially born through my experience exclusively pumping for my son.

This revised edition of *Exclusively Pumping Breast Milk* draws on my experiences pumping for my son and breastfeeding my daughter. Since the first edition was published I've accumulated another ten years of research, completed a course in breastfeeding support, had the pleasure of communicating with hundreds of exclusively pumping women, and perhaps even gained a bit more of the wisdom that comes with age. All these elements come together to create a more complete resource for pumping mothers.

It has been a genuine pleasure over the past ten years to support other women who are exclusively pumping and to share both my knowledge and experience. These women truly are heroes. They are inspirational and show the true meaning of love and dedication as they selflessly give of themselves to provide "expressed love" for their babies.

The book covers a lot of ground and ideally you'll want to read it from the beginning to the end. But if you're in a rush to get started, you may consider beginning with "Exclusively Pumping 101", "Pumps and Kits, Oh My!", and "Feeding Baby". These chapters will provide you with the basics. If you have a baby in the NICU, you'll want to ensure you read "Pumping and the NICU", in addition to the other three chapters, if you want quick access to information that will get you started. The book's index is also a handy way to help locate information or to find answers to specific questions you might have.

As you begin reading the book, I hope one thing is made clear: long-term exclusive pumping is possible. You will not be alone on your journey. I'll be here, as will many other women around the world who are, along with you, providing "expressed love" for their babies.

I would love to hear from you! If you'd like to share your successes—or need some emotional support—feel free to get in touch. You can connect with me through the book's Facebook page at www.facebook.com/exclusivelypumping or the book's website at www.exclusivelypumping.com.

Stephanie Casemore
May 2013

Introduction to the First Edition

Throughout my pregnancy I planned on breastfeeding. I knew that I wanted to give my baby the best I possibly could, and for me that meant providing breast milk for as long as possible. Around the beginning of my third trimester, I began to read books on the subject of breastfeeding to ensure I was prepared and knowledgeable, but having the time to read the volumes of information I collected was not to be.

Thirty weeks into my pregnancy, I developed severe preeclampsia and was immediately admitted into the antenatal ward of the hospital. Within four days of being admitted, I was induced and a few short hours later my tiny three pound, two ounce baby boy was born. Thankfully, he didn't have any serious complications other than his low birth weight, and, with the intention of giving him the best I could, I began using a breast pump since he was too small to nurse.

Initially, pumping was only intended to initiate my milk supply and ensure that I could breastfeed once my son was ready. Three weeks after his birth, I began short attempts to breastfeed him, and surprisingly, he seemed eager and ready. However, even after joining him in the hospital around the clock for almost two weeks, he was not strong enough to take full feeds at the breast and continued to be fed by a nasogastric (NG) tube, which is a tube inserted through the nose and placed directly into the stomach.

By the time he was thirty-seven weeks gestational age, we decided to introduce a bottle in order to get him home. Hospital policy stated that a baby could not leave the Neonatal Intensive Care Unit (NICU) until he or she was able to take all feeds by mouth for a 48-hour period. The importance of bringing our baby home before he fell ill in the hospital from the many viruses and bacteria lurking there was mentioned to me a number of times by different nurses. And so three weeks before his due date, we introduced the bottle and brought our tiny baby home.

Once home, life became an endless cycle of breastfeeding, bottle feeding to ensure he was receiving enough, and then pumping. On a good night, I was able to get four hours of sleep, although rarely four consecutive hours. Having been told to wake my baby every three hours to eat, I was quickly running on empty. Our breastfeeding efforts quickly deteriorated into extremely stressful experiences. My son would wail anytime I attempted to bring him to breast. He would scream and thrash and refuse to latch on. Needing to feed him, I resorted to bottle feeding in order to supplement our "failed" breastfeeding attempts. Throughout this, I continued to pump.

Eventually, in an effort of self-preservation, I decided that I would pump exclusively and feed by bottle. Once this decision was made, the stress level in the house dropped dramatically. Everyone, including my dog, seemed a little less on edge. But now I was faced with a future tied to a breast pump and no-where to go for support or information about exclusively pumping.

The internet became my best resource, and I located a number of discussion boards frequented by women who were also pumping for their babies. Suddenly I was no longer alone, and I realized it was possible to pump long term. These women became my source of information since they were doing it and proving it could be successful. At that time there were no available resources dedicated to exclusively pumping, and women had to figure it out for themselves. Not only did the internet provide much needed support and camaraderie, it also provided a valuable forum for women who were exclusively pumping to share their experience and techniques.

I continued to work with my son to develop a latch that did not rely on the use of the nipple shield that we had begun to use while still in the hospital. A couple of weeks after his due date we had success, put away the shield, and continued our efforts. Although I did not transition over to breastfeeding exclusively, my son did continue to breastfeed occasionally, often as a comfort measure and sometimes just because he was hungry. Complications of nipple soreness on my part and severe reflux on my son's part (which was not diagnosed for a number of months), as well as his preference for the bottle nipple, prevented a transition to exclusive breastfeeding. And so I pumped, happy to do it for the health of my son. I am grateful, however, that I was able to experience some aspect of breastfeeding although not the breastfeeding relationship I had expected. I exclusively pumped for just over one year and weaned by choice. After I weaned, I had enough frozen milk to feed my son expressed breast milk for another couple of months.

Exclusively pumping is an option! However, many women are not aware of it or are told that it is rarely possible and that they will not maintain a supply with a pump. While it is true that not every woman will see success, many women will, and obtaining good advice about exclusively pumping is the best way to achieve this success.

I am not a medical professional or a lactation consultant, but I did exclusively pump for one year and had to research and educate myself about lactation and pumping in order to pump long term. It is my intention to provide you with the valuable information I have learned in order to help you make an informed decision about pumping. I also hope to enable you to both establish your supply and maintain your supply for, hopefully, as long as you would like to provide breast milk for your baby.

The information in this book is also based on the generosity of over 50 women who took the time to share with me the method by which they started to pump and how they maintained their supply. It is their experiences which show this is an option available to many.

It is difficult to argue that breast milk is not the best nutrition possible for our babies. When breastfeeding just doesn't work out—either you cannot breastfeed, or do not want to breastfeed but still recognize the value of breast milk—there is an option other than formula. Women need to know this. You need to know this. While it is sometimes a more difficult road to travel, it is one that will be worth the effort when you look into the eyes of your breast milk-fed baby.

Stephanie Casemore
July 2004

Chapter 1

The Alternative to Formula

When my son was born, I was surprised by how emotional the experience was. I was suddenly responsible for a new life, and it was the choices I made that would determine, to a large extent, my baby's health and physical and emotional development. I was also surprised by just how exhausting a venture it was to be a new mother, but I was determined to push through the difficulties and provide the very best for my child. Let's face it, this is what mothers do. Our vision and focus immediately shift upon the birth of our first child: no longer are we the centre, but our baby becomes the sun in our solar system. Having a premature baby, with all the stress that naturally comes with it, and having a stressful, difficult experience trying to establish breastfeeding, I found myself at a crossroad: do I persevere and continue working to establish a breastfeeding relationship with him or do I make a choice to exclusively bottle feed him?

Formula was never something I thought I would feed my child. It was just not an option I had ever considered, and yet when I encountered breastfeeding difficulties, suddenly I was facing this possibility. Due to my son's early arrival in the world I had been pumping since he was born in order to establish my supply, and I decided that this is what I would continue to do. At the time, I didn't know if it was possible. I didn't know if other women did it. I just knew that breast milk was the choice I wanted to make for my son and I would give it to him any way I could. So began my experience exclusively pumping.

What is Exclusively Pumping?

Regardless of the paths that women may take to arrive at the option of exclusively pumping, the main definition is the same. Exclusively pumping, or exclusively expressing, often shortened to "EPing", means that a mother is expressing her breast milk and feeding her own expressed breast milk to her baby by bottle. Most women who exclusively pump use a breast pump to express milk; however, some women have even found long-term success using only hand expression techniques. Usually, the baby is exclusively fed by bottle, but sometimes a mother may also continue to nurse her baby, although most feeds are done with a bottle. While it is possible to initiate and maintain a full milk supply through exclusively pumping, some women do use formula supplementation if their supply is not fully meeting the baby's needs or if circumstances prevent her from pumping enough to meet her baby's needs.

Biological Expectations, Breastfeeding, and Breast Milk

Mother's milk is remarkable in its ability to provide what a child needs and more remarkable in its ability to change as a child grows, providing the optimal nutrition for that stage of a child's life. The living aspect of breast milk ensures that an infant's development follows the normal patterns for human growth. The overall composition of breast milk is specifically designed for human infants, and formula will never match its quality. And yet, is it true that "breast is best"?

The "breast is best" mantra has taken the maternal world by storm. Every new and expectant mother has read it and been taught it during pre-natal classes, in pregnancy and baby magazines and books, and by her doctor. Everywhere you look breastfeeding is declared as best for a child and for the mother. And indeed, breastfeeding not only provides optimal nutrition for the infant, it also provides long-term benefits for the mother. The World Health Organization recommends exclusively breastfeeding for the first six months of a child's life and continued breastfeeding for at least the first two years, continuing as long as mutually desired.[1] Most national pediatric associations recommend breastfeeding for at least six months as a minimum and many recommend a greater length of time. Large amounts of research money have been spent trying to fully understand the nutritional components of breast milk, and formula companies have continuously attempted to create a formula as closely resembling breast milk as possible. Of course an equivalent will never be created. But breast isn't so much *best*, as it is *normal*.

As biological beings, we have certain biological expectations. Breastfeeding is one of those. Babies expect to breastfeed and expect breast milk. They are born with the skills and reflexes to make this possible. Mothers, like babies, are also created to nurse their children. Aside from the obvious "equipment", mothers also have hormonal influences and skills and reflexes that make breastfeeding the fulfillment of biological expectations. Meeting these expectations, in a biological sense, affects our experience as mothers, and it ultimately affects children's experiences as they grow up.

Having said this, mothers make the choice that is best for their children, and sometimes this means pumping and feeding expressed breast milk by bottle, and sometimes it even means making the decision to feed formula. Regardless of the choice that is eventually made, it is important that a mother be well informed, and even more importantly, well supported, when making her decision. Often a mother is so stressed over the feeding of a new baby that everyone begins to suffer. Mothers feel overwhelmed, partners are unsure how to best support their spouse, and children experience the tension, anxiety, and frustration within the family. However, there is of course another option when a mother makes the decision to either stop breast-feeding or not to breastfeed at all: exclusively pumping.

The Alternative to Formula

Breastfeeding is by far the least complicated way to feed a baby. With no bottles to sterilize or warm and no formula to prepare, breastfeeding is practical and convenient for many. Having been able to breastfeed my second child for three years, I can un-equivocally state that breastfeeding is a wonderfully "lazy" way to mother. But from my experience with my son—twelve months exclusively pumping—I also know that breastfeeding doesn't always work out as expected and that this lost expectation can cause some very strong emotional reactions. (We'll talk about the emotional aspects of not breastfeeding in a later chapter.) When breastfeeding doesn't work out, or you choose not to breastfeed, the option that is most commonly presented is to feed commer-cially prepared infant formula, but exclusively pumping is an alternative that should be shared with new mothers. For those mothers who desperately want to breastfeed but who experience significant difficulties or due to circumstances are unable to breastfeed directly, the choice to exclusively pump can make the loss of a breastfeeding relationship a little easier, since it ensures that a baby can continue to receive breast milk.

The World Health Organization (WHO) recognizes a mother's own expressed milk as the next best option for infant feeding if breastfeeding is not possible.[2] Yet even with this WHO recognition of expressed breast milk, there has been limited research done on the use of a breast pump for long-term exclusive pumping or on the use and storage of expressed breast milk. Research, though, is slowly starting to surface, mainly conducted by breast pump companies and both non-profit and for-profit milk banks. There is certainly no doubt though that a mother's own milk is far superior—and closer to what is biologically expected—than artificial baby milk, or formula.

But while expressed milk may be closer to biological expectations than formula, exclusively pumping does not enjoy the same societal expectations and acceptance. The concept of exclusively pumping tends to be met with questions and misunderstanding. During my year of pumping, I remember a neighbour asking, during a power outage, why I couldn't simply put my son to my breast. And then there was the time I was asked by a family member why I couldn't just stop pumping for the two weeks I was on vacation and then resume when I returned home. Knowledge and understanding can sometimes be hard to come by. The reasons for pumping, and the process and time commitment involved, are equally misunderstood.

But indeed, a mother who chooses to exclusively pump should be lauded for her great efforts. For not only is she bottle feeding, with all the additional work that is attached to it, but she is also producing the food that she is feeding and pumping—sometimes eight to ten times a day to ensure her child gets the best she can provide. Frequently, women who exclusively pump do not feel it was a decision they made but, instead, that it was the only option they had left. As more women choose the option of exclusively pumping as an alternative to formula, it will become more understood and accepted.

Get Your Support in Place

Making the choice to exclusively pump requires support. Unfortunately meaningful support is not always readily available. Many well-meaning people have told women considering exclusively pumping that it is not a long-term option and that it is difficult to maintain your milk supply for an extended period with just a pump. While it is often true that a well-latching and efficiently breastfeeding baby is better at establishing and maintaining a milk supply, the number of women who have been able to exclusively pump successfully suggests that it *is* possible and it *is* an option. Yet even though mothers are doing the best they can for their babies, some people look upon the decision to exclusively pump in a negative way. They believe that it is a disservice to a baby and that every woman can breastfeed with enough dedication and effort. This attitude is one that forces some women to give up entirely and switch to formula, feeling inadequate for not being able to breastfeed.

The effects of stress and fatigue on a new mother are often overlooked or pushed aside in the attempts to establish a successful breastfeeding relationship. Sometimes, however, it is important to recognize that the mother needs to be healthy and functional in order to care for her child, and sometimes this will mean that the decision to stop breastfeeding may be a necessary one. Additional difficulties such as post-partum depression or family turmoil can, in and of themselves, create a difficult environment and the added stress of breastfeeding difficulties can become too much to handle.

Some people will also push the other way, stating that formulas are now excellent replacements for mother's milk and that the stress of trying to establish breastfeeding or exclusively pump is not worth it in the long run. While it is true that many babies do fine on formula, there is no formula that matches the exceptional qualities of breast milk.

In the end, the option to pump exclusively is often not presented at all to new or expecting mothers, but it is an option that needs to be shared. It is an option that people who work with new mothers must be aware of in order to fully support women and babies.

When looking for support, look for a professional who is knowledgeable, supportive, and preferably someone who has had experience assisting other women through the process of exclusively pumping. Do not rely on advice that does not recognize exclusively pumping as being separate from breastfeeding in terms of maintaining and establishing supply. While the goal is the same—to provide breast milk—the requirements to establish and maintain a supply exclusively with a pump are very different than simply pumping occasionally while breastfeeding. Many lactation consultants recognize the needs of exclusively pumping mothers and are more than able to support you.[3] But support doesn't only come from professionals.

Pumping can often feel like a very lonely road to travel. The first few weeks are tough and many women go through periods when quitting is constantly on their minds, but as every woman who has exclusively pumped or is currently exclusively pumping will tell you, it gets easier! Seek out support from those who will support your decision, those who will be there for you emotionally, and those who can assist you to work out the logistics. Seek out others who are pumping, whether they are in your community or on the internet. The internet provides many online discussion boards dedicated to those who are exclusively pumping. Surround yourself with support and keep focused on the reasons for doing what you're doing.

Exclusively pumping can be a viable option when you get accurate information and the support you need. It can help you provide the nutrition that is biologically intended for your baby: mother's milk.

Why Do Women Exclusively Pump?

The reasons for exclusively pumping are as varied as the women who exclusively pump. One thing all women have in common, though, is their desire to provide breast milk for their babies. Whether the decision to exclusively pump is made by choice or out of desperation, due to an ill baby or the perceived loss of other options, the ability to exclusively pump allows women to feed expressed breast milk for longer than they would otherwise be able to feed breast milk and allows them to forego the use of formula. Many women end up exclusively pumping when breastfeeding doesn't work out for them; this can happen for a multitude of reasons. A large number of women also come to exclusively pump when their babies are born prematurely. For this group, pumping is a necessity if they wish to breastfeed, and, in some cases, breastfeeding difficulties due to the many challenges a premature baby must overcome make it difficult to transition to exclusive breastfeeding. A mother may then choose to continue pumping long term. And of course, prolonged illness and the separation of mother and baby can make breastfeeding impossible whereas pumping can allow the baby to still receive the goodness of breast milk.

Prematurity

Almost every woman who delivers a baby before the thirty-fourth week of gestation must enter into the realm of pumping if she wishes to breastfeed her baby. Before the thirty-fourth week, a baby often does not have the strength or ability to latch and feed at the mother's breast. Once breastfeeding attempts begin, it may take a number of weeks before the baby is strong enough and has the required coordination to breastfeed effectively. It's important for mothers of preemies to initiate their supply with a pump and maintain their milk supply in order for their baby to transition to breastfeeding if possible.

Pumping for a preemie is in many ways different than pumping for a full-term baby. With a premature infant, the hope is usually that the baby will eventually be able to be put to breast and indeed breastfeed exclusively. While this is a possibility, and many women are successful at getting their preemies to breastfeed, there are also many women who are not able to breastfeed their preemie for a variety of reasons. Often, the mother of a preemie will feel that providing breast milk for her baby is about the only thing that she can do for her baby while he is in the hospital and, even when breastfeeding is not an option or proves challenging, providing breast milk can establish a connection between mom and baby. In the NICU, an environment that often feels very foreign and isolating, being able to provide expressed milk for your baby is something that only you can do as a mother.

Latch Problems

While breastfeeding is biologically expected, it does not always come easily. Interventions from society and the medical system, as well as a lack of support, can interfere with a mom and baby's breastfeeding relationship. Occasionally, a baby may develop problems with latch which make it difficult to continue to breastfeed. Concerns include a baby who will not latch, a baby who has a shallow latch, a baby who is sleepy and difficult to wake, structural concerns such as cleft palate or tongue tie, and a painful latch. While it may be possible to correct many of these problems, accurate information or support is not always available, and often the baby's health or a lack of weight gain necessitates a change, or at least supplementation. Of primary importance is the health of the baby, and if the baby is not eating well, then weight gain and dehydration become a very real concern. A mother's first concern is, of course, the health of her baby, so bottle feeding often becomes the method of feeding in order to ensure the baby is able to eat satisfactory volumes. At this point, a mother must decide what will be in the bottle.

Although there are methods of feeding a baby other than using a bottle and nipple (such as a Supplemental Nursing System (SNS), finger feeding, or cup feeding), bottle feeding is usually the most common method used when a baby needs to be supplemented or fed in an alternate way. It is, of course, also possible to turn to bottle feeding for a short period while you continue to work on the latch. Just because a baby has been given a bottle does not mean that baby will never breastfeed. However, it is possible for a baby to develop a preference for the bottle nipple since the flow is often faster and the baby does not have to work as hard to receive the milk. Still, it is possible to get a baby back to breast even at two or three months of age. Sometimes a baby just needs to get stronger in order for things to work out. So if you are unable to breastfeed from the beginning, but really want to, don't give up.

Sometimes, women who exclusively pump will continue to breastfeed their child simply for comfort as opposed to nourishment. This often will allow for the closeness of breastfeeding even though the bottle is still the primary vehicle for feeding. This option of continuing to breastfeed in a limited manner can ease the feelings of loss experienced when a mother is unable to breastfeed exclusively. In these situations, often a baby is able to latch but will not nurse long enough to take a full feed or perhaps has become accustomed to bottle feeding and no longer nurses when hungry.

If your baby has latching problems, it is extremely important to seek out the advice of an expert in the field of lactation. A board certified lactation consultant (IBCLC) will observe a breastfeeding session, diagnose problems, and can provide excellent advice on how to solve these problems. With the right strategies in place, many issues can be overcome and a satisfying breastfeeding relationship established. However, if you decide that you can no longer breastfeed, exclusively pumping is a viable alternative to formula.

Illness

Illness, of the mother or the baby, can lead a woman to exclusively pump. Anything that limits the contact of mother and baby will put a successful breastfeeding relationship at risk. A baby that is too ill to nurse will require alternative feeding methods and may be able to be fed breast milk by either bottle or nasogastric (NG) tube.

The illness of the mother makes the possibility of exclusively pumping more difficult, but, depending on circumstances, it may be possible. As with any other reason to exclusively pump, all the options must be weighed and a realistic look at the requirements must be taken. Depending on the mother's illness, exclusively pumping may not be possible due to the strict schedule required at the outset or medications that the mother is taking; however, it is worth discussing this option with medical professionals including a lactation consultant and medical doctors. Ultimately, the decision will be made by you in consultation with your medical advisors.

The illness of a baby may create a number of barriers to breastfeeding: hospitalization, lack of strength, or inability to eat orally resulting in the requirement of a tube for feeding. In all these situations, mothers desire to provide the best for their child, and breast milk is often seen as a way to provide the best. Pumping for an ill child can be extremely taxing on a mother who already has many additional stresses in her life due to the baby's illness. But, on the other hand, exclusively pumping for that child can provide the mother with a sense of empowerment, allowing her to nurture her child in this special way.

Separation

When mother and baby are separated for long periods, breast-feeding, of course, becomes extremely difficult. By pumping, the mother can provide breast milk for her baby even though she cannot be with the child. Nursing can continue when possible, and by pumping, the mother can maintain her supply.

Separation from your baby will require careful attention to the collection, storage, and transportation of the expressed breast milk. Depending on the distance you need to travel, this may be more challenging, but it is possible. Verse yourself in the safe storage and handling of expressed breast milk and determine the best possible methods for your particular situation.

Choice

Some women turn to exclusively pumping by choice. They have determined prior to giving birth that they do not want to breastfeed, but they want to provide the biologically normal source of nutrition for their baby—breast milk. The reasons for this choice are varied. Some women simply do not like the idea of a baby sucking at their breast. Many have to return to work soon after the birth of their baby and exclusively pumping seems like a plan that will still allow the baby to receive breast milk. Other women may have been sexually abused and have diffi-culty separating the abuse from their bodies. And some women may feel that exclusively pumping will provide them with more freedom than breastfeeding would. Regardless of the reason, the choice to exclusively pump will provide an alternative to commercially prepared formulas.

If you decide to pump from the beginning without attempting to breastfeed, be sure your doctor and the hospital staff are aware of your wishes. Ensure that your spouse or the person who will be with you during labour and delivery is comfortable standing up for your choice and is willing to make your wishes known to the staff. Research the availability of breast pumps in the delivery ward and, if necessary, bring your own pump with you. You may need to have your own pump cleared through the hospital building/electrical staff before using it, so find this out ahead of time.

Surrogacy

An often overlooked group of exclusively pumping women are surrogate moms who continue to nourish their surrogate babies after delivery by expressing their milk and providing it to the baby's family. Sometimes the baby is located nearby, but often surrogate moms who exclusively pump ship their milk a significant distance. While babies obviously benefits from surrogates' dedication and love, surrogates are also able to remain connected to the baby and continue to support the family—a truly selfless act.

Exclusively pumping may not be the road you wanted to travel, or it may be a conscious choice you've made, but regardless of the reasons you have come to exclusively pump, one thing is consistent: mothers choose this option out of love and a desire to provide breast milk instead of formula. While formula may sometimes still be necessary to supplement if enough breast milk isn't available, the love and dedication of a pumping mom can never be questioned.

Chapter 2

Making the Decision

Before committing yourself to the idea of exclusively pumping, it is important to be fully prepared for the ups and downs that may come along with the decision. Breastfeeding is an emotional issue. As mentioned in the first chapter of the book, breastfeeding is a biologically expected activity and when we do not breastfeed we sometimes feel loss, regret, or sadness. Breastfeeding is a relationship, and if you aren't able to have the relationship you expected some very strong emotions can surface. The emotions that accompany breastfeeding difficulties and the emotions that surround exclusively pumping are often closely connected and it is important to be prepared to work through them. It is also important to have a realistic picture of what the decision to exclusively pump entails. For some women, the ability to feed breast milk to their baby will far outweigh any negatives attached to exclusively pumping. However, most women who exclusively pump, at some point, will find the daily requirements taxing and question whether this is something that will be possible long term. (It most certainly is something you can do long term, and we'll talk about that soon.) The support of family and friends is also vitally important. Exclusively pumping takes up more time than other options and can affect the daily lives of your loved ones. And, as with anything, it is important to be aware of all your options before you commit. By being as well informed as possible, you increase your likelihood of success. My intention in this chapter isn't to dissuade you from making the decision to exclusively pump or to make it seem like exclusively pumping is a difficult, thankless and impossible task, but instead to provide you with an honest look at what it will take and what you might face in the months to come. So in determining if exclusively pumping is an option that will work for you, let's delve into these areas a bit more, explore what life is really like when exclusively pumping, and help you make an educated decision.

The Emotions of Breastfeeding and Not Breastfeeding

As if being a mother wasn't emotional enough, having to make a decision about how to feed your child when breastfeeding is no longer an option can bring to the surface many strong emotions. If breastfeeding was something you really wanted to do and something you looked upon as a bonding experience with your baby, the loss of this relationship may hit you very hard. And this is completely normal! Breastfeeding is a relationship and it is to be expected that the loss of this relationship will be something that you need to work through, grieve, and come to terms with. (For a much lengthier discussion on the emotions surrounding breastfeeding — and not breastfeeding — you may be interested in my other book *Breastfeeding, Take Two*.)

Many moms report going through a grieving period when they are no longer able to breastfeed. However, the opportunity to continue feeding your baby breast milk can help to ease this sense of loss. The feelings mothers report often centre on inadequacy and a feeling of failure. In fact, many women, when discussing their switch to exclusively pumping, will state that breastfeeding was a "failure" or that they "failed" at breastfeeding. It often takes time to overcome these emotions and talking to other women about your experience can be a great help. We'll discuss these feelings of failure, and the guilt that often goes along with them, in the next chapter.

Nearly every mother I have talked to admits to having feelings of guilt and loss over not breastfeeding. Breastfeeding is often seen as something that is uniquely part of a mother's experience; it is what we do. Other possibilities are often not even considered until the day you are confronted by the fact that breastfeeding is not working out as you had expected. Coming to terms with not breastfeeding can take some time. Taking it as a personal failure may be a natural response—but be kind to yourself. Taking on personal blame isn't changing the situation and in most cases doesn't reflect the reality of the situation. Focus on the facts and on the positives:

- A mother trying to cope under an increasing burden of stress is eventually going to break, whether it is her emotional or physical well-being that suffers.
- A baby needs his or her mother.
- The maternal bond is much more than the method of feeding.
- Even though you are not breastfeeding directly, your baby is still benefiting from your breast milk.
- Mothering is filled with guilt—this won't be the first thing about which you feel guilt! Focus on what you can control and what is going well in your life. Don't let guilt consume you.

- It is often possible to continue to breastfeed for comfort, if not to return to breastfeeding exclusively.
- Once you see how well your baby does receiving your breast milk, your decision will be much easier to accept.

It is important to remember that you need to take care of yourself in order to take care of your baby. During the process of making the decision to begin exclusively pumping, many women are completely overwhelmed. They are extremely sleep-deprived, possibly in pain due to thrush or a poor latch, frustrated, and feeling inadequate. All of this only increases the stress that new moms are feeling.

Seeking out the support and advice of professionals such as doctors or lactation consultants can be extremely helpful, but be prepared for the possibility that this will put more pressure on you either to continue to breastfeed, persevere through the problems you are facing, or else to switch to formula. Sometimes people think about the good of the baby but forget about the good of the mother. While breastfeeding can be good for both, the stress and strain of trying to establish breastfeeding can quickly take its toll and leave you with nothing left to give your baby. Only you can determine how much you can handle and how long you want to continue with your breastfeeding efforts.

Weigh your options carefully and objectively. Ask yourself these questions:

- How long can you continue as you are now?
- How much support do you have to continue breastfeeding?
- How much support do you have if you decide to exclusively pump?

- Have there been other extenuating circumstances surrounding the birth of your baby that have added to the stress you are feeling (e.g. illness, prematurity, c-section)?
- How will you feel in a few months about your decision if you stop breastfeeding?
- Are there any other avenues of support that you can use?
- Is your baby thriving?
- Are you constantly concerned about your baby's well-being and her ability to take adequate feeds?

While it is possible to get your baby back to breast if you stop breastfeeding for a while, it is more likely that you will not return to exclusive breastfeeding—so you need to be comfortable with your decision and prepared for the emotions you may experience. I think it is fair to say though that if you aren't able to breastfeed and you choose formula feeding over exclusively pumping you will still feel some strong emotions as a result of that choice.

As with any choice you make in life that does not follow the "norm", you will find no shortage of opinions from others about your decision to exclusively pump. A common experience among women who choose to exclusively pump is the confrontation of people who do not understand your decision. Many will say that it is impossible to exclusively pump long term and that you will never maintain your milk supply. Some may say that you are doing your baby a disservice by not breastfeeding. And yet others will tell you that you might as well switch to formula since it would be easier. There will always be someone who will question your decision, but in the end it is you who needs to be comfortable with it. So ignore the naysayers! On the other hand, you will meet people who will respect and admire your determination and commitment to exclusively pump for your baby. These are the people you want to keep close!

The Realities of Exclusively Pumping

Depending on when you talk to a mother who is exclusively pumping, she will tell you it's the hardest thing she has ever done or that it is simply part of her daily routine and can allow for some added freedom in her life due to the fact that others can feed the baby. The truth of exclusively pumping is that it can be a roller coaster of emotions, but, as every mother will also tell you, it gets easier.

Switching to exclusively pumping from breastfeeding is often done because you are completely overwhelmed trying to establish breastfeeding, experiencing difficulties such as a poor latch and ineffective milk transfer. Ironically, the decision to switch to exclusively pumping will not necessarily remove the feeling of being overwhelmed, but it can allow you to see a light at the end of the tunnel and allow you to refocus on solving any lingering problems. Having to pump frequently—and around the clock—can be extremely tiring. Pain caused by a yeast infection will not go away just because you decide to pump. A painful latch will not necessarily transfer over to a problem with the pump, but if your nipples have been traumatized, they may be sensitive to the pump as well.

However, most women find that exclusively pumping is an option that is possible long term. They no longer see their baby unhappy and frustrated at breast; they are completely aware of how much their babies are eating and are able to see them thrive; since others can help in the feeding of the baby, it is possible (although not always practical) that mom can get some extra sleep; and since baby is still receiving mother's milk and not formula, mom feels good about the nutrition her baby is receiving.

Once you get into the routine of pumping, it becomes just that—routine. However, exclusively pumping is more work than either breastfeeding or formula feeding. In fact, in many ways it is a combination of the two—and their challenges. Be aware of this before you start. Not only does it take time to pump (usually about two hours a day of pumping) but it also takes time to clean and sterilize bottles and pumping equipment—as well as time to bottle feed your baby. I'm certainly not saying this to frighten you, but it is important to go into the experience with knowledge and understanding of what you'll experience. But for all the challenges you may face, I think it is important to mention that I've never heard a woman say she wishes she hadn't made the choice to exclusively pump. The gifts of pumping, for both you and your baby, often eclipse the challenges.

The extra work and time commitment involved with exclusively pumping usually diminish as you go along. Whether you just get used to the schedule or completely forget what it would be like with the extra time in your life, it does get easier.

What to Expect

There are a number of things that almost every woman who exclusively pumps can expect at some point on her journey. Here they are, both the positive things to anticipate and the challenges for which to be prepared:

Things to look forward to:

- Looking into the eyes of your breast milk-fed baby and knowing that everything you are doing will benefit your baby for years to come
- Feeling a sense of pride and accomplishment
- Experiencing respect for your dedication and effort to feed your baby breast milk

- Having the opportunity to have others feed the baby
- Supporting biologically normal health and cognitive development for your baby
- Supporting biologically normal health for yourself as a result of lactation.

Challenges to prepare for:

- Lack of sleep (not that this is exclusive to moms who pump, but pumping will take more time away from sleep)
- Sore nipples and breast pain (this doesn't have to be a foregone conclusion, but be prepared for it because it can happen—although it is often because of improper equipment or pumping techniques)
- Misinformed people and people who want to know why you are not breastfeeding—yes, people can be nosy and opinionated!
- Feelings of resentment towards your pump (in the early weeks and months many women feel "attached" to their pump—physically, not emotionally—but this will pass)
- Difficulty juggling a baby and a frequent pumping schedule (there must be some law about babies that when the pump turns on, baby screams!)
- Overwhelming desires to quit (everyone has been here; you are not alone).

For information on how to overcome the challenges, see the chapter "You Can Do It! Overcoming Challenges".

Know Your Options

Most people, if asked, would state that there are two options for feeding a baby: breastfeeding and artificial baby milk, more commonly known as formula feeding. There is, of course, the third option to exclusively pump. It is important that you understand all of your options before making the decision to exclusively pump and to go into the decision with as much knowledge as possible.

If you are currently breastfeeding, but thinking about exclusively pumping, consider the other options you have before you:

- You can continue to breastfeed.
- You can switch to formula.
- You can seek professional help from a lactation consultant to assist you in establishing a successful breastfeeding relationship.

As previously mentioned, exclusively pumping is demanding and a lot of work. For most women, breastfeeding will be less effort. If you are considering exclusively pumping because you think it will be easier, less work, or allow you more time for yourself, please reconsider. If you do not want to continue breastfeeding full-time, there is always the option of pumping in addition to breastfeeding. This will allow you some freedom to go out, work, or sleep and have your partner feed the baby, but will also allow you the flexibility to breastfeed when necessary or desired, provide you with the hormonal connections derived from breastfeeding, and continue to provide your baby with most of the benefits of direct breastfeeding—not to mention the ability to breastfeed your older baby to calm them or soothe them, which is an incredible weapon in a mother's arsenal!

For those women who are having difficulty establishing breastfeeding for whatever reason, the ability to pump can allow you to maintain your supply until you can solve whatever is causing the difficulty. Pumping will keep your options open and give you greater flexibility. Consider getting advice and assistance from a lactation consultant; your local hospital or health unit should be able to connect you with someone who can meet with you and your baby and troubleshoot the situation. You may also find private practice lactation consultants listed in the Yellow Pages under "Breastfeeding" or "Lactation". Or you can try to locate a certified lactation consultant (IBCLC) through the International Lactation Consultants Association (ILCA) website, www.ilca.org. While not every problem can be solved, nor is everyone able to last under the stress of the situation, it is a good idea to work with a lactation consultant. It is worth seeking assistance with breastfeeding before choosing another road. If you are interested in a couple of techniques for returning your baby to breastfeeding, see the end of chapter 8, "Pumping and the NICU".

And of course, in every situation, the other alternative is to feed artificial baby milk. While some will say that it is an acceptable alternative, the honest statement is that it is the best alternative *if breast milk is not available*. The World Health Organization actually recognizes it as the fourth option for feeding a baby, with direct breastfeeding being first, a mother's expressed milk second, and donor milk from another source third.[1] Breast milk is by far the best nutrition for infants. Breast milk is living. It is able to change to meet the needs of your baby and pass immunity to your child. It is the easiest for a baby to digest, and provides the exact building blocks that an infant requires—not just for his current needs, but for his future needs as well.

Having said that, the success of formula companies today tells us that people are feeding their infants formula. Artificial baby milk has its place. It can be a lifesaving intervention and there are circumstances where it is needed—and thank goodness we have the ability to access it.

It is a fact that breastfeeding is not something that every mother will choose. If you are faced with this decision, you owe it to your baby and to yourself to be well informed. Gather as much information as you can about breast milk and formula. Educate yourself and make an informed decision. Most moms who choose to exclusively pump do so because they believe that breast milk is the best food for their baby, and they are willing to go the extra mile to provide it.

Making *Your* Decision

Now that you know the reality of exclusively pumping—the negative aspects as well as the positive ones—you will need to decide. The decision is yours to make. Trust your instincts. Don't allow yourself to feel guilty about making the decision. Don't allow others to force their will upon you. *You* are your baby's mother, and your baby needs *you*. You need to make the decision that will be right for both of you. This decision is different for every woman, and it is made for different reasons. You may perhaps continue to breastfeed. You may decide to switch to formula. You may decide to exclusively pump. Whatever decision you make, the decision should feel right and allow you to enjoy your baby, knowing that you are doing what is right for her.

Chapter 3

The Emotions of Exclusively Pumping

Mommy guilt. Every new mother feels it. It creeps in uninvited sometime during the first few weeks of your baby's life. It is unavoidable and, in many ways, it is a sign that you are a good mother. Perhaps guilt is a signal that you love your child. You want to do everything you possibly can for your child; you want to give her the best. Who can fault you for that? Yet when you've gone through a stressful or challenging experience and have not been able to meet your expectations for motherhood and caring for your child, guilt can sometimes hit you early and hard. If you are exclusively pumping by choice, then this is likely not something you'll experience, but for those who are exclusively pumping because of challenges breastfeeding or an experience that was outside of your control (premature delivery, cleft palate, health issues) it is likely that you will at some point struggle with feelings of guilt. When the worry—the belief that you are somehow harming your child or not providing them with what they need—begins to overwhelm you or becomes all consuming or ever-present, mommy guilt has reached a new level. A mother who experiences difficulties with breastfeeding often becomes consumed with a sense of guilt: a belief that she has let her baby down, that she has not given everything she could to her baby. "Guilt" is the name women will commonly give to the emotion they are feeling. Discussing the use of the word "guilt" Diane Wiessinger, in her essay "The Language of Breastfeeding", suggests it is an ineffective and inaccurate word, pointing the finger directly at a system that isn't doing what it needs to do:

> "We don't want to make bottle-feeding mothers feel angry. We don't want to make them feel betrayed. We don't want to make them feel cheated." Peel back the layered implications of 'we don't want to make them feel guilty,' and you will find a system trying to cover its own tracks. It is not trying to protect her. It is trying to protect itself. Let's level with mothers, support them when breastfeeding doesn't work, and help them move beyond this inaccurate and ineffective word.[1]

So is it really guilt? Do we really feel guilty when we are unable to meet our breastfeeding expectations?

Guilt vs. Grief

Guilt is something that comes at us externally. It is based on the judgment—or perceived judgment—of those around us. We are afraid of judgment from those around us, or else know that there is reason for us to be judged, and this causes feelings of guilt. Perhaps for some women feelings of guilt are proper and deserved; however, my experience communicating with hundreds of women over the past ten years has been that while women often name these feelings as guilt there is something else going on. In most cases, what women are feeling—in my opinion—is more accurately described as grief rather than guilt.

Guilt is something we feel when we know we could have done more, but didn't; when we went against our better judgement and made a choice we knew wasn't the best for those involved; or when we blatantly make a decision that we know is only in our own best interest and not in the best interest of those who we are to care for and love. Yet almost every exclusively pumping woman I've ever met has pumped because of breastfeeding challenges and a desire to provide her baby with what she believes is the best—breast milk. Where is there room for guilt? While 'guilt' may often be the word used to describe their feelings, 'grief' is perhaps a more accurate term.

The distinction between guilt and grief is not based on the amount of effort you put into breastfeeding or the length of time you persevered. It really has more to do with the information you had at the time, your efforts to access information and support, and your dedication to do everything you could do *at the time*. Once you have exhausted your resources—and for some, those resources are going to be very thin—you have a decision to make. If you are faced with a baby who is hungry, who is not gaining weight, or who is crying incessantly, you need to feed your baby. Without the resources and support to help you breastfeed successfully, what else are you going to choose? You choose to bottle feed, whether it is expressed breast milk or formula in the bottle. When you have exhausted your resources, and done all you can do, there is no reason to feel guilty. As new mothers, we do what we believe is right at the time. There is no guilt in that.

On a very personal level, I understand this sense of guilt all too well. When my son was born so early and so tiny, the guilt set in. My body had failed him. I had developed preeclampsia at thirty weeks and he was showing signs of intrauterine growth restriction. The day before I was induced, doctors tested the umbilical blood flow and determined that it was in the ninety-seventh percentile. This high percentile was not a good thing and meant the blood flow in the cord was compromised. My son was doing okay, but my body was quickly shutting down and the doctors determined it was best to deliver right away. My determination was then to ensure I could breastfeed. I remember asking several times during a quick tour of the NICU what the chances of breastfeeding were. Would I be able to breastfeed my son? All indications were positive, and so I clung to that hope. My body wouldn't fail my son again.

But five weeks later, even though my son was doing very well with expressed milk and I was determined to make breastfeeding work, it was not working. Feelings of failure were strong; I figured I just didn't know what I was doing. The lactation consultants in the hospital seemed frustrated that my son was not breastfeeding better than he was, and I internalized this frustration, thinking I was the cause. As I left the hospital for the first time with my son, I remember feeling emotionally numb. I was operating largely on auto-pilot and still clinging to the belief—the hope—that breastfeeding was going to work out.

Of course, life rarely goes as planned and things got progressively worse at home. Eventually, it got to the point where he was projectile vomiting several times a day, screaming after most feedings, and thrashing and wailing if I attempted to latch him. It became very personal. Was my son rejecting me? I sought out assistance from lactation consultants and breastfeeding experts. The advice ranged from "It's okay to switch to formula if that is what you want" to "You've got to get that baby to the breast" but with no offer of help or useful suggestions. After finally resigning myself to exclusively pumping, partly to preserve at least a small degree of my sanity and partly as a retreat from defeat, I found one doctor who suggested a diagnosis of reflux and offered a readily available, over-the-counter medicine to see if perhaps it might help my son. In less than twenty-four hours it was as though a new baby had moved into the house.

Guilt? You bet! But I quickly realized that I had done everything I could do with what I was given. I had lactation support in the hospital. I sought out lactation support when my son was released from the hospital. I talked to my doctor. I demanded a referral to a pediatrician. I read the books. I searched online. I was screaming for help; and yet the system—or perhaps more accurately, society—failed me. What more could I have done? Could I have continued trying to breastfeed exclusively? Possibly. But if you have gone through the cycle of breastfeeding, pumping, and bottle feeding you understand what an incredible toll that takes on you. It is not a long-term solution. Could I have stopped pumping and just breastfed to see how well my son would have done if he was forced to breastfeed with no bottle in sight? I could have, but I felt at the time that all I had going for me was a strong milk supply and I feared I might risk it all if I stopped pumping. I felt alone and lonely in the experience. And in hindsight, I know that I did all I could do, physically and emotionally, to make it work. But still it didn't.

And so we're left with guilt and grief. Once you work through the feelings of guilt, and recognize that you have done all you could do given your knowledge, support, and physical and emotional limitations, you are left with the grief. Breastfeeding is a biologically expected activity. It is, for most women, a relationship that is deeply desired. To lose that relationship is to lose something very real, something that has value and purpose and meaning. Just as we mourn when we lose a person we love, we must also mourn the loss of the relationship we wished for.

Part of the challenge in understanding these feelings as grief, as opposed to guilt, is the way that breastfeeding is framed in our society. Many people surrounding you may have a "get over it" attitude. Many suggest to new moms who are having breast-feeding difficulties, "Just switch to formula." But these attitudes and well-intended suggestions serve only to make us feel that our emotions are wrong and that feeling sad over our loss is invalid—but it most definitely is not! Working through these emotions is critical, both to your well-being and your baby's well-being. Coming to terms with your shared, rocky start will help you grow and move forward.

Moving Forward

Regardless of what we call it—guilt, grief, or regret—the experience of losing the breastfeeding relationship you had hoped for and expected can, and most likely will, affect you in the future. It may hide in a corner or be an obvious stumbling block in your decision to have other children. It may appear to have been tamed and controlled, only to unleash itself when you get that positive sign on the pregnancy test. The impact of breastfeeding failure can be varied, but for most women who experienced difficulties breastfeeding, the impact is very real.

Grieving takes work. It also takes time. But you can help yourself by identifying your feelings, examining them, and working to accept them and move forward from your experience.

First, it is important to take some time to reflect on what you expected. What expectations did you have for the process of breastfeeding? How were those expectations met or not met? It's natural to have expectations about things, but having expectations without flexibility can lead to an increased sense of loss. When you only picture one possible outcome, there is nothing but disappointment and loss from any other outcome. When faced with an experience that is not what you expected, it is necessary to comes to terms with it. It is the shared, developing relationship between you and your child that is most important. Exclusively pumping may not what you expected, but it is yours.

When breastfeeding doesn't go as expected, there is a true loss for both mother and baby. As mothers, we lose out on what we planned for and hoped for, and both we and our babies lose the natural process and bonding relationship fostered by breastfeeding. It is so important to recognize it as a loss and allow yourself to grieve the loss. It's okay, normal even, to be sad. Often those around us don't recognize the loss or understand why we feel so sad. If you're feeling overwhelmed and have no one to talk to, consider finding a doctor or therapist to whom you can voice your emotions. Do not bottle up your feelings, or push them away, thinking that you're overreacting. It *is* sad when a mother and baby lose the opportunity for a nursing relationship, and working through your emotions will help you put your experience in perspective.

The next important step is to recognize the experience for what it was. Everything we do is a learning experience. We don't always have all the answers; no one should expect us to. But we do have the opportunity to learn from our experience and move forward with intention. Once you're feeling capable of honestly looking at the reasons breastfeeding didn't work out, try to pinpoint what it was that went wrong. Consider the three big elements: lack of information, lack of support, and societal pressures and influence.[2] Where did it go wrong in your case? Be clear here. This is not intended to be a blame game. The idea isn't to find blame in what you did or didn't do. We all do the best we can, with the information we have, at a given time. But to move forward, we need to be able to look critically at our experiences and actions and understand what happened.

The grief you feel is deeply personal and is something that you alone need to work through. Jessica Restaino considers this personal aspect of grief and breastfeeding in her essay "Drained" in the book *Unbuttoned*, explaining, "In many ways that's what getting better was like. It was a breaking away from something deeply personal, deeply mine."[3] This "deeply personal" aspect of breastfeeding is felt by almost every mother. It's our biology that creates it and yet it's our culture that defines it. If our society tells women that they are being ridiculous for being so emotional when they are unable to breastfeed, then mothers are left feeling badly about the sadness and grief. Restaino states that her "sadness became a source of guilt."[4] It is so important to recognize your emotions for what they are—sadness, grief, anger, guilt...whatever they may be. Accept them as your own, work through them, and then, most importantly, figure out a way to move past them.

Once you've grieved the loss and examined your experience and hopefully better understand what happened, the last steps are to reframe your experience in a positive way and then move forward with intention. While you may never look back on your breastfeeding difficulties with fondness, they are part of your story, your experience. They have added to the person you are today. Perhaps your experience has given you greater empathy, encouraged you to search out new ways to bond with your baby, or brought you new friends you may not otherwise have met. Your difficulties have certainly helped you understand the level of your own persistence and drive, as well as your own limitations. Considering what you have gained, and not just what was lost, can help you move forward with purpose.

Don't Overlook What You Have Done

The dedication required to exclusively pump, regardless of how or why you arrived there, is awe-inspiring. It is not an easy feat, but then again, neither is being a mother! If you are grieving the fact that you were unable to breastfeed, recognize that your attempt to breastfeed shows your care. Your determination to try and make it work shows your love. Your willingness to push through the pain and discomfort testifies to your dedication. If you did all you could given your circumstances, then there is no room for guilt. Regret, yes. But not guilt. Grieve, move on, and learn from your experience.

If your experience is not what you expected, don't overlook the incredible thing you are doing and be sure to recognize the amazing commitment and strength you are exhibiting. Watching your baby growing because of your milk—whether you are able to provide 100% of your baby's nutrition requirements or not—is an incredible thing. *You* are doing that—no one else! Just as you nourished your baby in your womb, you are continuing to nourish him or her outside your womb. And the nourishment will continue. Once you wean your baby from your milk, the nourishment just takes a different form, relying more on love, compassion, guidance, and gentle discipline.

It's easy to point out the ways we feel we have let our children down: things we should have done, or did but shouldn't have. Mommy guilt. This is always going to be part of motherhood. So you weren't able to breastfeed your baby. That is a terrible loss, and one that you need to grieve and move forward from, but it's not the sum total of your value as a mother. Remember to keep it all in perspective. You love your baby, and you do everything possible to give your child the best you can. Sometimes as parents we don't do so well, and other times we are awesome! This is life. Breastfeeding is just another aspect of mothering. It's worth fighting for, and it is wonderful when it works out, but it does not define you as a mother, nor does it define your relationship with your child.

Chapter 4

Lactation and Breast Milk Composition

Ιn order to successfully pump long term, it is important to have a basic understanding of lactation and the composition of breast milk. While it is not essential to have extensive scientific knowledge, it is helpful to have a general sense of how things happen. There are many books already published that go into great detail about the structures of the breast and the process of lactation, so this *won't* be a master class on the subject. Rather in this chapter we'll look at the basics of lactation and gain an understanding of the key factors in breast milk production which will enable you to make informed decisions when it comes to exclusively pumping. I do encourage you to search out as much information on this topic as you can. The more you know, the better prepared you'll be. When breastfeeding, it is easy to rely on your baby's instincts to manage lactation—when your baby is hungry, you nurse—but when exclusively pumping it is up to you to set the schedule and create the demand so your supply will be sufficient for your baby's needs.

Critical Factors in Milk Production

An understanding of the lactation process is important for all mothers. Understanding how lactation is initiated and regulated can help you establish a strong milk supply, maintain that supply, and make decisions that reduce any potential negative effects on your supply.

Stages of Lactation

Lactogenesis I begins during pregnancy. The mammary glands change from inactive to active preparing for lactation. About half-way through pregnancy, the breasts will begin to produce colostrum. You may or may not experience leaking at this time. Breasts usually enlarge, veins become darker, the areolas enlarge and darken, and the nipples become more erect.

Lactogenesis II begins following the detachment of the placenta. This stage of lactation is triggered by a sharp decline of progesterone following the detachment and subsequent delivery of the placenta. Any retained placenta can greatly affect a mother's ability to establish a full milk supply.

Formula provided during this time (even just once) changes the normal flora of the gut and it can take days for it to return to normal. The gut flora of a breastfed baby is significantly different from that of a formula-fed baby.

Milk production slowly increases over the first few days postpartum. It usually takes two to five days for milk volumes to increase, but it can take longer depending on a variety of factors such as certain birth interventions or medical conditions. First-time mothers will see an increase later than mothers who have already had children.

It is important to realize that lactogenesis II will happen regardless of whether a woman is choosing to nurse her baby, express her breast milk, or formula feed her child since lactogenesis II is a result of hormonal factors.

Stages of Breast Milk

There are three stages of breast milk:

Colostrum is present at birth and is all a baby requires until milk production increases. It is yellow to orange in colour and is very thick and somewhat sticky. Colostrum is high in antibodies and protein and has a laxative effect, which assists a baby in removing meconium from her system. If meconium is not removed from a baby's system, it can lead to jaundice since bilirubin from the meconium will be reabsorbed. Colostrum also coats the gut providing protection from potential pathogens. It's important to realize that a baby's environment is sterile until birth. Once born, a baby is suddenly exposed to a host of dangers. Nature has provided the initial dose of colostrum as an "inoculation" against these many dangers. Since the mother has already been exposed to these dangers in the environment, her colostrum will provide antibodies against those elements specific to her environment.

If pumping, it is important to collect and feed colostrum, not only for the laxative effect, but also its immunological elements that will assist your baby in fighting off infections. While some pumping mothers choose to supplement with formula at birth, this is not always necessary, depending on how long it takes your milk to increase. Colostrum will assist the baby's digestive system to begin its work, rather than being pushed into high gear immediately at birth.

Transitional milk follows colostrum. It can be seen as early as twelve hours after delivery—although usually takes longer—and usually lasts one to two weeks. It is the consistency of mature milk, but it retains some of the colour of colostrum.

Mature milk has a slight bluish tinge to it and is rather thin when compared to formula or whole cow's milk. It contains all the nutrition that a baby needs for at least the first six months of life. Breast milk will continue to change throughout lactation, responding to the needs of the infant, the mother's exposure to viruses and bacteria, and the mother's diet.

The Hormones Involved

Prolactin

Prolactin is the hormone responsible for triggering milk production. It is also referred to as a "mothering hormone" because it creates nurturing responses. Prolactin levels rise sharply following delivery and fall substantially over the first twenty-four to thirty-six hours post-partum. Prolactin is produced by the anterior pituitary gland and causes a decrease in estrogen levels. It also inhibits the maturing and release of eggs from the ovaries. The absence of menstruation during lactation is known as lactational amenorrhea. Prolactin levels naturally vary throughout the day with the highest levels in the early morning hours between 1a.m. and 5a.m. Once lactation is established, prolactin takes on only a permissive role as opposed to a regulatory role: it no longer drives production but its presence simply allows milk production to continue. While there has been no research showing a correlation between serum prolactin levels and breast milk volume, it is necessary to maintain prolactin levels for its permissive role.[1] Prolactin and dopamine have an inverse relationship. As dopamine levels rise, prolactin will decrease. If you have a condition or take medications that raise dopamine levels, this may cause issues with lactation. Smoking is one common activity that will raise dopamine and smoking has been shown to have a negative effect on lactation.

Likewise, it is important to note that progesterone may interfere with normal prolactin production and its interaction with cell receptors.[2] Progestin-only (mini-pills) birth control is the best oral contraceptive to use while lactating; however, due to the possibility that it may interfere with the establishment of the milk supply, it is usually recommended that you wait until your supply is well established before starting even progestin-only birth control. Oral contraceptives containing estrogen are not recommended for lactating women. Seek the advice of a knowledgeable physician who is experienced with lactation and the possible effects of birth control. If you do take hormonal birth control and find that your supply is starting to decline, stop immediately and use a different form of birth control.

Oxytocin

Oxytocin is vital during both the birthing process (contractions) and lactation (milk ejection reflex). It is also a "loving hormone" assisting in creating affection and social bonds with others. Oxytocin can help to create a relaxed, calm, and euphoric feeling, which both the mother and the baby experience when breast-feeding. Oxytocin is important to the bonding of mother and baby and, in the presence of prolactin and its influence on mothering responses, oxytocin helps to create a strong bond between mom and baby. Oxytocin levels in the brain soar immediately after delivery—this is one reason why immediate and uninterrupted one-on-one time following a baby's birth is so important. Unfortunately, when pumping, the release of oxytocin is not associated with the connection between mom and baby. However, oxytocin is not only released during breastfeeding (or pumping) but also when we share meals together, hug or kiss, or share close connections, and so you can still build a strong bond with your child, even when not directly breastfeeding.[3]

Oxytocin receptors in the breast increase during pregnancy and also increase in the uterus prior to delivery. The uterus uses oxytocin to prevent post-partum hemorrhages by contracting the uterus. Oxytocin is released from the pituitary gland when the nipple is stimulated. Just as with breastfeeding, mothers may experience after-pains when pumping in the days following delivery.

Oxytocin acts upon the smooth muscles of the breast and causes contractions which push the milk into the ducts and to the nipple. The milk ejection reflex, or let-down, takes place multiple times during a feeding or pumping session since the oxytocin is released in waves as stimulation continues. As a new wave of oxytocin is released, a new let-down will occur. This knowledge is important for the mother who is exclusively pumping. Many women will stop pumping once their milk flow has slowed, having been told they should pump only a few minutes after the flow of milk has stopped. However, since the milk ejection reflex is initiated by waves of oxytocin being released, the flow of milk will also come in waves. It may take two or more let-downs in order to remove a sufficient amount of milk from your breasts.

Once lactogenesis II has begun, milk production is largely controlled by the baby, or in the case of a woman exclusively pumping, controlled by the pump and frequency of pumping sessions.

Endocrine and Autocrine Control

The production of breast milk is dynamic and active, and the control of production changes over the first few weeks postpartum. The breast responds to the stimulation of an infant or pump with a series of events that release hormones, which in turn stimulate a milk ejection reflex, or let-down, and prompt further production or signal the breast to decrease production if, for some reason, the milk is not removed from the breast.

Endocrine control refers to the hormonally driven stage of lactation—lactogenesis II—which will happen regardless of whether a baby is nursing or not (with rare exceptions such as Sheehan's Syndrome or physiological conditions such as hypoplasia) and which lasts for a few weeks after a baby's birth. During this time, lactation is established and supply is set. Milk production will vary depending on the amount of stimulation to the breasts, nipples, and areolas, and the frequency of stimulation. This is an amazing aspect of nature since the variation in frequency helps a mother regulate her milk supply depending on the number of babies she has. So milk supply will be different for the mother of a single baby as opposed to the mother of twins, and when exclusively pumping this must be taken into consideration. For this reason, it is vitally important that when pumping you pump frequently.

Autocrine (local) control is also referred to as lactogenesis III and is the maintenance stage of lactation. This relies on the principle of supply and demand, and it is both interesting and important to know that milk synthesis is controlled at the breast and independently in each breast.

So there are then three things necessary to maintain breast milk supply:

- there must be the required hormones present and they must successfully travel to the breast (known as endocrine control);
- there must be stimulation to the nipple, areola, and breast; and
- the milk within the breast must be removed (known as autocrine control).

Two Key Processes Controlling Milk Production

Milk removal is the primary control mechanism for milk supply. In other words, milk removed from the breast initiates more production of milk in the breast. As the scientific community continues to research lactation, the understanding of milk production continues to develop. One of the most important things to understand about lactation and milk production is this: milk production slows as the breast fills. This is a central tenet of milk production.

Far too often I read or hear women telling other women that perhaps they are not waiting long enough for their breasts to "fill up" again in between pumping sessions and this is why they don't have enough milk. This well-meaning advice goes against everything science teaches us about the process of lactation. If you want to produce enough milk you must pump frequently and remove as much milk as possible from the breast. Milk left sitting in the breast slows production. There are two reasons for this:

> 1) A mother's milk contains a protein called Feedback Inhibitor of Lactation (FIL). As the breast fills, naturally more FIL is present and production will begin to slow. Think of this process as a grocery conveyor belt. As you put groceries onto the belt, you have less and less room to add more groceries and eventually you must stop adding items because you have run out of room. In order to allow more groceries to be added—or breast milk to be produced—you must remove some of the groceries—or milk. Anyone who has ever suffered from engorgement will appreciate this little protein. It is important to have some limits on production or else engorgement, plugged ducts, and mastitis would be far more prevalent than they already are.[4]

> 2) When the alveoli (small sacs that contain milk-producing cells) are full of milk, their walls expand and the shape of the prolactin receptors changes. (You'll remember that prolactin is the hormone that both initiates lactation and allows lactation to continue.) This prevents prolactin from entering at

these sites and, as a result, slows milk production. As the alveoli empty, the receptors return to their normal shape, allowing prolactin to enter again and milk production to increase.[5]

These two processes are key to understanding milk production. Both frequency and efficiency of milk removal are primary in the initiation and continuation of production. Anything that interferes with these two aspects has the potential to interfere with or harm the continuing lactation.[6] It is clear that when milk is removed more frequently, then production will increase.[7]

The Prolactin Receptor Theory

The prolactin receptor theory is another important idea in lactation and has implications for all pumping moms. The basic idea of the prolactin receptor theory is that milk production is "set" during the first few days and weeks post-partum. Frequent stimulation increases the number of prolactin receptors in the breast, allowing the body to utilize prolactin more effectively. This sets milk production for the rest of the lactation period. Newborns naturally feed for short periods but feed very frequently. This encourages the increase of prolactin receptors and the establishment of a strong milk supply. For mothers who are using a breast pump to initiate their milk supply, it is important to understand the prolactin receptor theory and to follow a pumping schedule that provides frequent stimulation and removal of milk.

The most important aspect of the prolactin receptor theory is that the newborn's seeming desire to breastfeed all the time is biology's way of ensuring the mother's milk supply is ample five months or more down the road. Even though it may seem that there is no milk in the breast and that a baby is getting "nothing", a newborn who is nursing frequently is getting exactly what is needed and ensuring that will continue as he or she grows and develops. Hospital practices that separate mom and baby, birth interventions that prevent a baby from nursing within the first hour following delivery, or early bottle supplementation all have an impact on this natural process and interfere with the normal development of prolactin receptors that are critical to long-term breastfeeding. As a pumping mom, this means that you also want to pump frequently and follow nature's plan as closely as possible.

Storage Capacity and Milk Production

Storage capacity is the amount of milk the breast can hold between nursing or pumping sessions. Storage capacity is *not* directly related to the size of the breast and can differ between breasts; in fact the right and left breast rarely produce the same amount of milk.[8] Storage capacity also has been shown to change during lactation.[9] Storage capacity of the breast affects the rate of milk production.[10] A large storage capacity will allow milk production to continue for a greater length of time before slowing since the receptors will not "stretch" until full. Think of this concept as a cup: you can drink a large amount of water throughout the day using any size of cup. If you use a small cup you will simply have to refill more often.[11] This is not an indication that a woman with a larger storage capacity can produce more milk, only that a woman with a smaller storage capacity will need to nurse, or pump, more frequently.

For a breastfeeding mom, storage capacity may affect a baby's feeding pattern. Mothers who have a smaller storage capacity will likely have babies that nurse more frequently. This is important for both the mom's milk supply and for the baby's sufficient intake. Mothers who have a larger storage capacity may have babies who go a little longer between nursing sessions, depending on the amount of milk a baby wants when nursing. A baby whose mother has a large storage capacity will more likely feed from only one breast when nursing as opposed to nursing from both breasts during each feeding.

And what does this mean for a mom who is exclusively pumping? Just like a nursing mom who will need to nurse more or less frequently depending on her storage capacity, moms who are pumping will also be lead by their individual storage capacity to some extent with regards to how frequently they need to pump. Although when initiating supply it is important to pump frequently, once milk supply has been established a mother with a larger storage capacity can often drop to fewer pumping sessions than a mother with a smaller storage capacity and still maintain her supply. Unfortunately, there is little you can do to thwart nature and you're stuck with the storage capacity you've been given.

Research has shown, however, that the storage capacity of breasts increases between one month and four months post-partum.[12] This is particularly heartening for women who have struggled with production in the early weeks. Many women do find that production will continue to increase with good pumping habits over the first two to three months post-partum and perhaps this increasing storage capacity plays a role in that. While milk production is not dependent on breast volume (i.e. the amount of breast tissue), the study does suggest that both do naturally decrease over time. Apoptosis, which is a process of cell death that is programmed to occur, begins to happen around six months and breast tissue begins to involute; however, milk production continues. Decreased prolactin plays a role in apoptosis, and decreased frequency of milk removal, which results in milk left sitting in the breast, can also encourage apoptosis. For this reason, frequent expression should be continued for as long as possible when long-term pumping is your goal. The good news is that while storage capacity is related to milk production, there is no such connection between breast volume and milk production.[13] Whether A cup or DD cup, it doesn't matter.

Composition of Breast Milk

Breast milk is an amazing combination of fats, proteins, vitamins, minerals, growth factors, hormones, enzymes, and immuno-protective elements. While lactation will occur regardless of whether or not the mother is eating a well-balanced diet, the levels of certain elements in breast milk are determined by the mother's intake while levels of other elements are not. Carbo-hydrate and protein levels are not greatly affected by the mother's food consumption and tend to remain at a relatively constant level. However, the level of fats in breast milk can vary depending on a number of factors. Vitamin and mineral levels are also related to the mother's own intake. Breast milk has incredible bioactivity (the ability for it to affect living cells) and bioavailability (how easily it is absorbed and used). While a lactating woman should of course make every effort to eat as nutritiously as possible, poor diet should not be thought of as a reason not to provide breast milk.

The volume of milk a mother produces is not greatly affected by her diet. Milk production remains at a fairly constant level. In addition, increasing your intake of fluids will not necessarily increase your volume of milk. It is important to remain well hydrated; however, it is not necessary to drink excessive amounts of water or other fluids. In fact, over-hydrating can lower your milk supply. The best strategy is simply to drink to thirst.[14]

Fat Content in Breast Milk

The concept of foremilk and hindmilk is a rather outdated one. Research has shown that fat is released into milk as the breast empties.[15] Milk expressed from a full breast will have an increasing amount of fat as the breast empties and milk expressed from a less full breast will have a more consistent level of fat throughout the pumping session. The amount of fat in breast milk has been shown to have no relation to the frequency of breastfeeding, and we can assume this holds true to the frequency of expressing. Fat content does vary throughout the day with a higher level of fat during the day and evening and a lower amount in the morning and at night.[16] If you express when your breasts are very full , you will notice that the first milk is thinner and more watery, and milk that is expressed from a breast that is not exceedingly full will have a fairly consistent level of fat throughout the pumping session.

When pumping, especially if you have a strong supply, it is good practice to mix milk from a single session or even from a number of sessions to ensure the amount of fat is consistent. However, it is unlikely that a baby who is being fed expressed breast milk will experience what is often referred to as a "foremilk/hindmilk" imbalance. If you are pumping consistently and frequently, mixing milk from a session, and ensuring you empty your breasts as much as possible when you pump, your milk should have a fairly consistent level of fat.

A baby's intake, and *not* the amount of fat in breast milk, is the *only* thing that has been connected to infant growth. It is important to realize though that the type of fat in your milk is largely influenced by the type of fat in your diet. So do avoid the nasty trans-fats and opt for healthier unsaturated fats, omega fats and medium-chain fatty acids such as coconut oil. If you make a point of eating a wide variety of healthy foods, ensure you get sufficient calories, and minimize your intake of unhealthy fats, the composition of your milk shouldn't be a concern—and eating a healthy diet will give you the energy you need to keep up with the busyness of motherhood.

Specific elements found in breast milk:

Proteins
- not affected by the nutrition of the mother
- provide the baby with protection against pathogens through both specific and non-specific immune responses. Non-specific responses are those that do not require previous exposure to the microorganism in order to do its job (e.g. digestive enzymes, phagocytic cells which ingest bacteria). Specific immune responses require exposure to the pathogen (e.g. antibodies, lymphocytes).

Fats
- greatly affected by the nutrition of the mother
- also affected by length of gestation, length of lactation, number of children mother has had, and weight changes of the mother
- mothers of premature babies will produce milk that has a higher fat content and it will stay at higher levels for the first few months of lactation
- weight gain during pregnancy has a direct correlation to a higher fat content in breast milk
- fat content increases as the breast empties
- the higher the volume of milk you are producing, the lower the amount of fat in that milk

Vitamins and Minerals
- vitamin and mineral levels depend on the mother's own vitamin and mineral status and you may consider taking a multivitamin daily

- vitamin D should be supplemented if daily sunlight exposure is limited, if you have a darker complexion, or you live in a northern location
- iron in breast milk is highly bioavailable, meaning even small amounts of iron are more readily absorbed than the larger amounts found in formula
- breast milk contains an element, lactoferrin, that binds with iron making it easier for the baby to utilize

Immune and Non-immune Protecting Properties

- the production of these protective elements relates closely to the baby's own ability to produce their own immunity
- as the baby's own immune system begins to work independently, the protective properties of breast milk start to change
- during the baby's gestation, and during her first few months of life, the mother provides passive immunity to the baby (transfers immunity through the blood stream and then through breast milk)
- passive immunity is extremely effective for the first six months or so of a baby's life. After this time, the space between the cells of the baby's small intestine "closes" making it more difficult for the relatively large antibodies and other proteins to pass through into the baby's blood stream.
- the immune properties of breast milk have been shown to reduce the incidence of necrotizing en

terocolitis, diarrhea, respiratory infections, otitis media, diabetes, lymphoma, Crohn's disease, and urinary tract infections
- also contains antiviral, antiprotozoan, and anti-bacterial properties
- increased immune function in breast milk-fed babies can be seen not only when they are receiving the milk, but for several years after weaning
- it also may be that the immune systems of breast milk-fed babies mature more rapidly than their formula-fed counterparts

Growth Factors and Hormones
- growth factors and hormones are essential for proper growth and development
- stimulate the production of blood cells and the maintenance and repair of tissue

Enzymes
- assist baby with functions that have not yet fully developed such as pancreatic functions and digestive functions

Biological Expectations and Breast Milk
Rather than talking about benefits of breast milk, it is more meaningful to talk about biology and biological expectations. As mammals, we are expected to breastfeed. That's why we have breasts! Thousands and thousands of years have brought us to a place where we, as babies, expect to be nourished at our mother's breast, and as mothers, we expect to nourish our babies at our breast. However, this doesn't always play out as biology expects.

Things happen. Societal attitudes and beliefs come into play. Information and support is lacking making it challenging for mothers to breastfeed. And in many cases, mothers have to return to work soon after the birth of their babies, which can make breastfeeding difficult. Sometimes exclusively pumping is the best option available. In an ideal world, every baby and mother would have their biological expectations met, but we don't live in that world. Recognizing these expectations is important, though, since feeding your baby in as close a way as possible to the expectations will ensure your baby's needs are met.

Breast milk is amazing in its ability to perfectly meet the nutritional needs of human infants. Breast milk is protective and its impact is long-lasting. Breastfeeding is the biologically normal method of feeding babies, but even when direct breastfeeding is not possible, or not desired, feeding expressed breast milk still ensures the biologically normal nutrition is received by our children—even if it is not the usual delivery method. But not only is breast milk biologically normal for babies, lactation itself meets the expectations of mothers, ensuring that key health and psychological needs are met.

Most research on breast milk investigates those babies who are breastfeeding. It is possible, in many instances, however, to transfer this understanding of breast milk to the breast milk-fed baby. Yet breastfeeding is not all about the milk. There is the element of nurture in addition to the nourishment. While all mothers strive to create a strong, personal bond with their children, the way you achieve a close bond when pumping may differ from breastfeeding mothers and babies. However, using certain feeding strategies and paying attention to the need for connection and closeness can enable mothers to meet the need for connection in other ways. We'll talk about some of those strategies in an upcoming chapter.

There are some aspects of breastfeeding that cannot be achieved when feeding expressed milk. If you are able to breastfeed, then that option will allow your baby to have all its biological expectations met. However, it is undeniable that feeding expressed breast milk remains a far superior choice when compared to feeding commercially prepared formulas.

How Do Direct Breastfeeding and Breast Milk Feeding Compare?

There is plenty of research that investigates the incredible qualities of mother's milk, and chances are you are already sold on the idea that breast milk is the way to feed your baby. In this section we'll consider the differences between direct breastfeeding and breast milk feeding (using expressed breast milk and feeding by bottle). Ultimately, breast milk is always going to provide elements that no manufactured infant formula will ever come close to. Breast milk is a living substance that is created for *your* baby, specifically offering protection against the environmental dangers to which *your* baby is exposed, yet many exclusively pumping mothers are concerned about what differences there really are between breastfeeding and expressed breast milk feeding.

For the purposes of comparison, we'll assume you are feeding freshly expressed breast milk. In most cases, the influence of breast milk will be the same for both direct breastfeeding and expressed breast milk feeding. If you are pumping from day one and are able to feed your baby colostrum, the colostrum will act as a laxative to clear meconium out of your baby's digestive system, reducing the risk of jaundice. As previously discussed, colostrum also lines the intestinal track, preventing pathogens from entering your baby's blood stream. Colostrum is a mighty boost of immunity, providing concentrated antibodies and protecting your baby from environmental risks.

Other areas in which your baby will experience effects similar to breastfeeding include the following:

- increased immunity and immune system maturation,
- reduction of risks from pneumonia, gastroenteritis, botulism, and bacterial meningitis,
- reduction of risks of chronic diseases such as lymphoma, Crohn's, celiac disease, ulcerative colitis, juvenile rheumatoid arthritis, and type 1 diabetes,
- reduction of risks of allergies, asthma, and eczema,
- support for optimal brain development,
- reduction of risk of necrotizing enterocolitis, which is especially important for preemies, and
- protection against viral, bacterial, and parasitic infections.

That is quite a list and there are still some other ways breast milk may influence your baby. However, it should also be noted that, with some of these other benefits, it is not yet entirely clear what effects are due to the influence of the milk itself and what effects are actually related to the delivery method for that milk.

One such area is breastfeeding's impact on obesity later in life. The effects of breastfeeding on obesity are still disputed. If it does play a role in maintaining a future healthy weight, it is unknown what causes the correlation. One possibility is that breastfeeding allows a baby to self-regulate their eating whereas bottle feeding (regardless of what is in the bottle) tends to allow a baby to eat more and parents often encourage a baby to finish the entire bottle. The other possibility is that the components of breast milk themselves play a role in decreasing the likelihood of obesity later in life. While there may be some connection to the milk itself, research does suggest that the delivery method plays an important role in the development of obesity.[17,18, 19] To reduce the impact of bottle feeding as much as possible, it is important to bottle feed as you would breastfeed, which means watching your baby's cues, allowing your baby to control the process as much as possible, and using feeding time as a time to bond with your baby. For more information on how to bottle feed in this way, see the section on paced bottle feeding in chapter 9.

Another protective aspect of breastfeeding that can't be clearly connected to breast milk feeding is the reduced risk of Sudden Infant Death Syndrome (SIDS). The relationship between Sudden Infant Death Syndrome and breastfeeding is not entirely clear. There have been studies that show a small positive correlation between the two. However, other risk-reduction measures such as laying the baby on his back to sleep, removing any fluffy bedding from the crib, and parents not smoking are also of benefit. While it seems that breastfeeding does decrease the risk of SIDS, the reason for that is unclear. It is possible that the close contact between a mother and breastfed baby may reduce the risks. Breastfed babies have been shown to have a higher arousal level than their bottle feeding counterparts, although this may simply be due to the fact that more breastfed babies are co-sleeping or sleeping in closer proximity to their mothers. It is also a possibility that the reduced number of infections in a breastfed baby lowers the risk of SIDS. In the latter case, breast milk-fed babies should also see the benefit. Regardless of the mechanisms of SIDS, it is clear that keeping your baby in close proximity, ensuring no one smokes in the house or around your baby, keeping fluffy blankets and crib bumpers out of the baby's bed, and laying your baby on his or her back to sleep are all important steps in keeping your baby safe.

One argument you'll hear frequently regarding bottle feeding instead of breastfeeding is that breastfeeding provides a mechanism of bonding between mother and baby, and that breastfeeding allows for the close skin-to-skin connection that facilitates bonding. It is true that breastfeeding provides this, and any mother who has breastfed will attest to the close bond that develops between her and her child. However, breastfeeding is not the only way to bond with your child and when breastfeeding hasn't worked out as you've hoped, you shouldn't feel as though you'll be unable to bond with your child. Bonding has just as much to do with the connection between you and your child and your desire to interact with, and be present for, your child. Many bottle feeding mothers are exceptionally well bonded to their babies, and conversely, there are breastfeeding mothers who have not bonded well with their babies. You may grieve over the loss of breastfeeding and the relationship you had expected to have with your child, but do not feel that the relationship is lost or unattainable. It will simply be developed in other ways. Likewise, the benefits of skin-to-skin contact are entirely dependent on whether a mother chooses to practice skin-to-skin time with her baby. Skin-to-skin contact is not a benefit solely for breastfeeding; it can be experienced with a bottle-fed baby as well.

There are a few aspects of breastfeeding that do not readily translate to bottle feeding expressed breast milk. One is a baby's oral development. A mother's nipple, when latched onto by a baby, flattens and elongates. This helps to ensure proper oral development, especially of the palate. You can choose to use orthodontic-type bottle nipples, but Mother Nature did it best and it will be difficult to replicate the interaction between a mother's breast and a baby's mouth with a bottle and nipple. Breastfeeding also helps to develop hand-eye coordination in the infant. Since breastfeeding is bilateral and a baby is switched frequently from one side to the other, a baby develops its vision and hand-eye coordination from both sides. One way to mimic this when bottle feeding is to switch sides and not hold your baby in the same arm for every feed. Tooth decay is a final item of comparison with breastfeeding having the potential to reduce tooth decay. Breast milk certainly has some protective elements against tooth decay, but if a baby is allowed to take a bottle to bed, milk may pool in the baby's mouth and this may increase the risk of dental caries. This pooling of milk does not normally occur with breastfeeding babies. Ultimately, good oral hygiene is important and regular teeth cleaning should begin as soon as your baby's teeth come in.

A frequent question I receive from pumping mothers is regarding the interaction between a baby's mouth on the nipple, saliva, and immunity. There is a theory that suggests saliva will enter a mother's breast as the baby nurses. The pathogens in the saliva will then trigger the mother's immune system to manufacture antibodies against it, and these antibodies will then be shared with the baby through the mother's milk. While information about this potential immune pathway is limited, there is some research to suggest this may indeed be the case. What we do know is that our bodies gather information from a number of different pathways including the gut (Gut-associated Lymphatic Tissue—GALT), the respiratory tract (Bronchial-associated Lymphatic Tissue—BALT), and mucus membranes (Mucosa-associated Lymphatic Tissue—MALT). The mammary glands are part of the MALT system and contain lymphatic tissue. When a mother's immune system produces antibodies in response to an invading pathogen, the lymphatic system carries these antibodies throughout the body, including into the mother's breasts. Some cells that originate in the Peyer's Patches in the digestive tract actually stay in the breast and produce their own type of antibody which is then shared with the baby through breast milk. Likewise, any pathogen that may enter a mother's breast would be caught in this lymphatic tissue and would be transported through the circular lymphatic pathway to the gut where antibodies would be produced and returned to the breast and secreted into the milk. This combined system is known as the enteromammary immune system.[20]

So what does this all mean for a pumping mom? If antibodies are produced in the gut and the lymphatic system circulates antibodies throughout the mother's body, including the breast, then pathogens that you are exposed to within your environment will get passed along to your baby through your milk. It certainly is possible, however, that your baby is exposed to pathogens to which you are not exposed, especially if your child is in daycare or spends time in a different location without you. If breastfed infants do indeed pass pathogens from their saliva into their mother's breast tissue, then this is a direct communication that will not be available to a bottle feeding mom and baby in the same way it is to breastfeeding infants and mothers. Some suggest that mothers allow even a non-breastfed baby to suckle at the breast for a short period every day, or to take a small amount of your baby's saliva and put in on your nipples. However, it is unclear what mechanisms would allow saliva to enter the breast, if this type of communication does indeed happen. It may perhaps be just as effective to share lots of kisses and snuggles with your baby, allowing the pathogens on your baby's skin and saliva to be shared through this close contact. In the end, there is still a great deal we do not understand about lactation, immunity, and the properties of breast milk.

Breastfeeding has numerous health implications for a mother, not just for her baby. In almost all cases, the effects of breastfeeding on mothers are related to the hormonal profile of a lactating woman, and for this reason there is little difference between a breastfeeding mother and a pumping mother. The hormonal "benefits" of breastfeeding include the following:

- the release of oxytocin during the milk ejection reflex in the immediate post-partum period helps to return the uterus to pre-pregnancy size and decreases the risk of hemorrhages after delivery; afterpains are common when pumping in the early days after delivery

- as long as stimulation of the breasts remains frequent and continues during the night, there is often a delay in the return of ovulation and menstruation—but not always, so don't rely on it as a form of birth control
- due to delayed menstruation, known as lactational amenorrhea, there is a decreased risk of iron deficiency
- the increased caloric demands of lactation may cause easier weight loss in the post-partum period, although this isn't the case for every woman
- due perhaps in part to the low estrogen levels during lactation, the occurrence of breast cancer, ovarian cancer, and uterine cancer are lower in women who have lactated
- type II diabetes is reduced in mothers who have breastfed and would assumedly translate to exclusively pumping mothers
- lactation will actually decrease bone mass, possibly due to the infant's need for calcium, which is taken from the bones, or due to the decrease of estrogen, which is a hormone that protects the bones; however, the good news is that calcium is quickly restored after weaning, often within six months, and bones can be even stronger. There have been studies that show breastfeeding can reduce the risk of osteoporosis.[21]

And of course the health benefits for an infant who receives breast milk, both short-term and long-term, can't be overstated. While this may be seen as a good thing for babies, it is definitely a good thing for moms!

Post-partum depression may be reduced by breastfeeding, but there has also been a suggestion that breastfeeding difficulties may exacerbate post-partum depression. It stands to reason then that stress and challenges that lead many women to exclusively pump may in fact increase the risk of post-partum depression; however, if a new moms feels overwhelmed with breastfeeding challenges and finds the stress diminishes if she makes a decision to exclusively pump, then the risk of post-partum depression may again decrease.

Chapter 5

Exclusively Pumping 101: The Basics

It would seem that exclusively pumping should be quite simple. You have a breast pump and you have breasts; you would think that milk should be expressed and both you and your baby should be happy. While this can be the situation for some women, others will find it takes a bit more work—not to mention information and support—than would first be expected. But do not fear! Thanks to continuing research on human lactation and the mechanics of milk expression, and the many women who have found success exclusively pumping long term, there are "best practices" that you can learn from and follow to help you provide expressed breast milk for your baby.

Let's start first with a list of tips and "tricks" that you can quickly and easily put into practice. We'll then discuss the importance of the milk ejection reflex, specifics relating to how to establish your milk supply with a breast pump, switching to exclusively pumping after breastfeeding, maintaining your supply, supplementing with formula, and dropping sessions. If you want the quick introduction to pumping, this is the chapter for you.

Tips and Techniques

Aside from bringing the pump flanges to your breasts and turning on the pump, there are some useful guidelines and suggestions that will make your experience more productive and less tedious. Using these strategies and techniques will help you make the most of the time you spend pumping and help to increase your supply in order to meet your baby's needs.

- Double pump! Not only will double pumping save you time, you will also make the most of your prolactin levels by double pumping. Double pumping simply means expressing from both breasts at the same time. Be sure the pump you choose has the capability to double pump. Research is showing that the use of a double pump, as opposed to pumping only one breast at a time, yields results in terms of increased supply.[1]

- Use hand expression. Combining hand expression with double pumping can help to increase milk supply, especially if used in the early weeks when establishing supply. Try hand expressing at the end of your pumping sessions. This will help remove remaining milk, provide additional stimulation, and in the early days will help to express colostrum, which is quite thick and sticky and therefore often difficult to express with a pump. For more information about using hand expression, massage, and compressions when pumping please see the chapter "Pumping and the NICU" where it is discussed in more depth. Also, for a good visual explanation of how to use hand expression see the video produced by Stanford School of Medicine.[2]

- Hands-on pumping techniques (massage and compressions while pumping) have been shown to increase milk production, and one study showed a mean daily volume increase of 48%, so if you're not using your hands, what's stopping you?[3]
- Massage your breasts prior to pumping. The stimulation can assist you in achieving a let-down. Or you can try massaging your breasts while you are pumping. Some women find it helpful to lean forward while massaging.
- Use breast compressions while you are pumping. Hold your breast with your thumb on one side and fingers on the other and gently compress the breast closer to the chest wall and well back of the areola. Compressing on the areola can reduce milk flow instead of increasing it. Compressions will assist in getting out more milk and can both clear and help to prevent blocked ducts.
- Take a warm shower or use warm compresses prior to pumping. The warmth can stimulate your breasts and help to achieve an easier let-down. You can buy round gel pads that can be warmed (or cooled) and even worn while pumping.[4] For an inexpensive compress, pour some water into a newborn-size diaper and warm it in the microwave and then place it on the breast. Not too hot though!
- Ensure your nipples are centred in the flanges. If not, this can cause excessive friction and soreness.
- Enjoy lots of skin-to-skin contact with your baby, especially early on. Not only is this a nice, restful

and intimate time to share with your baby, it will also encourage your milk production. Many mothers find that they will pump more milk after snuggling with their babies. Consider wearing your baby in a carrier such as a sling, wrap, mei tai, or soft structured carrier.[5]

- Think of your baby while you are pumping. Attach a photograph to your pump. Watch your baby sleeping. Think of her adorable smile. This baby-body connection will assist you in letting down for the pump and help you to relax. We aren't meant to release milk for a machine, so it can take time to develop a good let-down, especially if you are transitioning to exclusively pumping from breastfeeding. Use the emotional connection you have with your baby to help elicit a let-down response.

- Use some type of lubrication to prevent excess friction. While not an absolute necessity, many mothers find the use of a lubricant beneficial in reducing any possible chafing and it will help keep your nipples soft. Options include lanolin, although it is important not to use lanolin if you have thrush. Some mothers choose to use olive oil instead of lanolin as lanolin may be a bit too sticky. Olive oil has some antibacterial properties and is much less viscous than lanolin. Another increasingly popular option is coconut oil, which also has antibacterial, antiviral, and antifungal properties.[6] This is also a good option if you have a yeast infection. Go with what works for you, but do consider some type of lubricant to prevent discomfort. Whatever you choose, be sure it is safe for your baby. While very little will find its way into the expressed milk, it is possible to have trace amounts.

- Get comfortable. You are going to be spending about two hours a day sitting and pumping. In the year I exclusively pumped, I calculated I spend about one entire month in direct "contact" with my pump! So with that much time sitting down, you want to find a comfortable place to do it. Ensure you are warm enough—or cool enough. Bring your phone close by or turn it off so you are not interrupted. Get yourself a glass of water or juice and place it within reach. Put your feet up and relax. If you fall asleep, you won't be the only woman who has done so while pumping. Read a book. Surf the net. Whatever you do, just be aware of your posture and any tension in your body. You don't want to create back or shoulder problems.

- Leave your pump set up in the location where you pump most frequently. Dismantling your pump, or putting it out of the way, will just add to the time it takes to pump. Pumping is going to be part of your life, so it might as well be out for all to see. My pump never left my living room for the entire year I pumped—it didn't matter who was visiting! If you want, throw a towel over the pump so it isn't as noticeable. Having it set up and ready to go will make it much easier to add in an extra session here or there if you are trying to increase your supply, or will simply make those early morning sessions quicker and less of a hassle.

- Relax! Sometimes this is much easier said than done; however, it is important that you relax when you are pumping. If you are stressed or tense, it can interfere with your ability to let-down your milk. Think of the time you are pumping as a mental health break. Allow this time to be time for you. Read a book. Enjoy a tea. Call a friend. Do not sit and worry about the housework or whether your baby is going to wake up from his nap before you are done (if you're lucky enough to be pumping while your baby naps). In the end, it's important to try to develop a Zen-like attitude towards life: it will all work out, things will get done, and right now you are focusing on what's important.

- As an extension of the above point, find something to occupy your mind: read, surf the internet, watch television, talk on the phone. Do not bottle watch! The old adage, "A watched pot never boils" is especially true when pumping. You will begin to worry that you are not getting much milk and this will in turn inhibit your let-down, which will make you worry more! Remember that oxytocin is necessary for a let-down, and oxytocin, as well as being called the "hormone of love", has also been referred to as a "shy" hormone.[7] When we are stressed, feeling unsafe or self-conscious, or fearful, oxytocin will often not make an appearance. This is sometimes seen in labouring women whose contractions mysteriously disappear once they arrive at the hospital and are suddenly inundated with noise and machines and people parading in and out of the room. Trust that it will happen as it should and enjoy your time doing something else.

- High suction alert! In general, you want to pump at the lowest suction level that removes milk for *you*. You will need to experiment to determine where this level is. Each pump will be different as well, so if you change pumps, do not rely on the control knob to indicate the amount of suction. Too high a suction level will damage your nipples very quickly and make it painful to pump, which in the end can reduce the amount of milk you are able to express.

- Check the size of your flange. Pumps come with a standard flange size, but let's face it, we're not all the same standard size! Using a flange that is too small or too large can affect your milk supply and cause discomfort. Flange diameters range from 21 mm to 40 mm. If you are experiencing sore nipples or areolas, or experiencing low milk supply, consider the size of your flange. You may need a smaller or larger one. If you are unsure, contact a lactation consultant or your local health unit and ask for a consultation. More about this in the chapter on pumps and kits.

- Go hands free—if you want. You can purchase pumping bras designed to hold the flanges in the bra, allowing you to use your hands for other things, such as massage and compressions or surfing the internet. Or you can make one yourself by taking a snug fitting bra and cutting slits in it to allow you to slip the flanges inside. Some women become extremely adept at balancing collection bottles on their knees, allowing them to use their hands, but a pumping bra makes this unnecessary. A quick internet search will yield a good number of results for hands-free pumping bras.

- Do not wear underwire bras or tight, constricting bras. These can cause blocked ducts and affect your supply.

The closer you can stay to the "normal" biological expectations of breastfeeding, the better things will usually go. So keep that in mind. There is sometimes the false assumption that a breast pump is a magical device that will wondrously maintain your milk supply on just a few sessions a day, but if a newborn baby is nursing eight to twelve times a day you should expect to pump just as often. And a baby wouldn't go six hours through the day without eating, so you too should not go six hours without pumping. Keep nature in mind as you proceed on your pumping journey. While we can't always match it exactly, it's worked for thousands of years.

The Milk Ejection Reflex

The milk ejection reflex (MER), or let-down, is the holy grail of pumping. Without a strong let-down, you will have greater difficulty establishing and maintaining a strong milk supply. The MER happens when a wave of oxytocin causes the cells around your alveoli to contract initiating the ejection of milk from your breasts. Women will experience the MER differently: some will never notice it at all, some will experience some slight tingling and a sensation of their breasts filling up, and some will experience what they would describe as mild pain or discomfort. It is also common for the sensation of let-down to decrease as time goes on. As with many things, it is very individual and there is a wide range of "normal".

Often the sight of your baby or the sound of his cry will initiate the MER when you are breastfeeding; however, when pumping this may not be the case. Your body will become conditioned to different things and you actually need it to become conditioned to initiating the MER when you are pumping. One interesting feature of oxytocin is that its release is dependent on environmental factors. Dr. Michel Odent refers to it as the "shy hormone".[8] When we are cold, stressed, feeling observed, scared, or threatened, oxytocin will not be released. Techniques mentioned earlier such as being relaxed, taking a warm shower before pumping, looking at a picture of your baby (or your actual baby for that matter), massaging your breasts before you pump and while you are pumping, and doing something while you pump other than watching your collection bottles and wishing they would fill faster, will all assist in experiencing easier, more effective let-downs. At the same time, feeling rushed, being in an unfamiliar environment, or worrying that someone is going to walk in on you will be counterproductive.

Since the MER is in many ways a conditioned response, try to maintain a similar routine when you are pumping: sit in the same location, do the same thing, listen to the same music. You will also want to limit, as much as possible, things that can negatively affect the MER including stress, fatigue, embarrassment, cold, pain, smoking, caffeine, alcohol, and some medications.

Most women will have more than one let-down per pumping session. This is important to know. Often, pumping mothers are told to continue pumping until milk flow stops or only drops are coming, but this happens once the let-down ends. This doesn't, however, mean that there is no milk left to express. By continuing to pump and adjusting the suction and cycling—as we'll discuss shortly—you will get multiple let-downs and remove more milk. While the first let-down usually nets the most milk, the additional sessions are important. Milk ejection patterns are largely individual and they are also consistent, so once you figure out your pattern of let-down, you should be able to count on it.[9]

The Darker Side of MER

The wave of oxytocin in your body during the milk ejection reflex usually brings with it a feeling of relaxation and calm. It's a "feel good hormone" that connects people and, for most mothers, the physical sensations of let-down are positive. Dysphoric Milk Ejection Reflex (D-MER), however, is a condition that causes negative emotions just before let-down and may last for a few minutes after milk ejection. Women experiencing D-MER may have sudden feelings of sadness, anxiety, or even anger. Although not common, it is important that women who do experience D-MER are aware of it and know that they are not alone.

D-MER is categorized as mild, moderate, or severe, based on how the mother perceives the symptoms, how long they last, during how many let-downs per feeding or pumping session it is experienced, and other factors. It is believed that D-MER is a result of a sudden and inappropriate drop in dopamine levels in the body. Dopamine and prolactin function are closely connected. In order for prolactin levels to increase, dopamine must decrease; however, in mothers experiencing D-MER, dopamine drops quickly and to an extreme low. The dopamine decrease is triggered by the rise in oxytocin that precedes let-down.[10] Once dopamine levels stabilize, the woman will feel fine; yet, the emotions experienced during the episode can be devastating and difficult to cope with.

The good news is that research is showing treatment can be effective for severe cases of D-MER. In some situations, D-MER can be managed with lifestyle changes such as stress reduction, exercise, getting adequate sleep, and using distraction during episodes of D-MER. Various natural treatments may also help including the use of B vitamins, acupuncture, and herbal supplements such as Rhodiola. For severe cases, prescription medications may be necessary. Bupropion, the active ingredient in Wellbutrin, appears to be the best option. It works as a dopamine reuptake inhibitor, which allows dopamine in the body to be used more fully.[11] For further information about D-MER, there is an excellent website maintained by a lactation consultant who herself suffered from D-MER before it was even recognized as a condition. The website is at www.d-mer.org.

Cycling and Suction: Finding a Pattern That Works

Cycling refers to the number of "pull and release" cycles per minute. Suction is the strength of the pump's draw. A breast-feeding baby will have a cycle rate of about 45-55 suck and release cycles per minute. A baby's suction level is about 200-220 mmHg when actively nursing. A baby's nursing pattern will, however, change depending on whether there is an active let-down or whether the baby is suckling to elicit a let-down. If you have breastfed, you'll recognize this pattern of quick, light sucks before milk starts to flow and then, once the let-down begins, longer and stronger draws as the baby actively drinks milk. Over time, you will discover a pattern that works best for you. Until you establish your own method, here's a good strategy to begin pumping:

When starting your pumping session, start with a low suction level and high number of cycles (this is assuming the pump you are using will allow you to adjust both, as some will not). If you have been breastfeeding, try to mimic your baby's sucking pattern. Once you start letting down, decrease the cycle speed and increase the suction. This pattern can then be repeated to achieve a second let-down, and perhaps even a third. Many women mistakenly stop pumping after the flow from the first let-down slows not realizing another let-down is possible.

To help women elicit a let-down there are breast pumps currently available that have this type of pumping program automatically built in. Pressing the let-down phase button will switch the pump to slower cycling and higher suction. While this may be a good feature for many women, pumps that allow you to vary the cycles and suction yourself are just as effective and allow you to individualize your pumping session. Ultimately, special features only matter if the pump is comfortable and effective for you.

If you find you have difficulty getting a second or third let-down you might try taking a break. After a let-down, when the milk flow slows, turn off your pump. Take a few minutes to grab a drink, check on your baby, put a load of laundry in the wash, and then return to the pump and finish your session. Some women find that this physical break is quite beneficial and a stronger let-down occurs once they take a short break.

Initiating Your Milk Supply by Pumping

Okay, so we've gone through many of the tips and techniques that can be helpful when pumping, but how are you actually going to establish your milk supply with a breast pump? What kind of schedule is necessary? What are the most important aspects of exclusively pumping? That's what you really want to know, right? Let's now talk about how to initiate your milk supply when exclusively pumping.

When initiating your supply exclusively pumping, frequency is critical and its importance cannot be overstated. You should aim to pump approximately every two hours, at least eight times a day, with one longer stretch in the night. It is important that you pump at least once between 1 a.m. and 5 a.m. since during this time your prolactin levels are at their highest. Your goal should be to pump *at least eight times* within a twenty-four hour period—extra pumping sessions are bonus.

It is important to begin pumping as soon as possible following your baby's birth. While it is likely impractical for you to express immediately following delivery, don't delay any longer than necessary. Remember that your prolactin levels spike immediately after delivery, so you want to begin pumping as soon as possible—and as frequently as possible—to benefit from those high levels.

It is not necessary to pump for extremely long periods during the first few days post-partum. Twelve to fifteen minute sessions will suffice. If you are pumping more than eight times a day, you can reduce this time to ten to twelve minutes. Remember that frequent stimulation is what is most important at this point. Try not to go longer than three hours between sessions during the day when initiating your supply and ensure at least eight sessions per day.

Until your milk increases in volume you will be expressing only small amounts of colostrum. It can take up to seven days or more for your milk to "come in" and certain birth interventions, such as excessive IV fluids, can cause a delay in lactogenesis II. Don't worry about the small amount of milk you are expressing in the early days! This is as it should be. Newborns require very little in the first hours and days of their lives. Be consistent and trust the process. What you are doing now will lay the groundwork for your milk supply in the months to come. This initial schedule is grueling. I know! But resist the temptation to cut back on sessions at this stage of pumping.

Do be sure to feed your baby what you are expressing. This first milk, colostrum, is extremely valuable to your baby. It can, however, be a bit difficult to express colostrum with a pump. After you pump use hand expression techniques to remove any colostrum still remaining in your breasts. You can hand express into a small collection cup or onto a small spoon and feed it directly to your baby. To feed colostrum that you have expressed with the pump, try using a small syringe (without the needle of course) to both collect the colostrum and to feed it to your baby.

You can, during this period, supplement with formula if you wish. However, remember that breastfed babies would not normally be receiving anything but colostrum from their mothers, and there is no need to supplement breastfed babies at this stage in their lives unless there are medical complications that require supplementation. Your baby will have the desire to suckle though, so if you are not breastfeeding you should consider the use of a pacifier, since a feeding bottle nipple will not sufficiently meet a baby's suckling needs.

As has been previously mentioned, once your milk supply starts to increase, continue to pump every two to three hours with at least one session between 1 a.m. and 5 a.m. A good schedule for the first few weeks is *eight times a day, for about fifteen to twenty minutes per session*. See the next section in this chapter on the length of sessions, frequency of sessions, and total amount of pumping time per day for more information on how long to pump.

As you continue to pump, gauge your schedule by your supply. You want to establish, if possible, a daily volume that slightly exceeds the maximum daily intake of your baby at his highest intake level. You may decide you want to have a very large supply, or you may need a larger supply if you are pumping for multiples. However, keep in mind that with a larger supply problems such as engorgement, difficulty weaning, and storage issues can sometimes arise. Unless you are only planning on pumping for a short amount of time and want to freeze as much milk as possible, you may want to prevent your supply from growing too large. While opinions will vary, I would suggest that volumes in excess of 1350-1500 milliliters/day or 45-50 ounces/day are unnecessary for most mother-baby pairs.

Considering that most babies' *maximum* daily milk intake will be around 960 milliliters a day (32 ounces) with the average intake being around 750 milliliters (25 ounces), a volume in excess of this maximum will rarely be required. Establishing a supply around 1200-1500 milliliters (forty or fifty ounces) will allow for ample milk to freeze and should cover any reduction in supply that may occur when dropping pumping sessions. But it will ensure you do not have too many issues with excessive milk storage, low fat content, or engorgement. Once again, all this is very individual. Some women will maintain a very consistent volume regardless of their pumping routine, while others notice significant decreases as they change their schedule. In my opinion, it is best to be prepared for decreases rather than worrying about not having enough expressed milk to feed your baby.

Some very interesting research recently conducted by Peter Hartmann's team in Australia suggests that a breastfeeding mother's supply is remarkably consistent from about four weeks to six months post-partum.[12, 13] From this, it can be assumed that a baby's intake during this time is also consistent. Babies who are receiving breast milk do not tend to increase their intake over the first six months of life as babies receiving formula do. Breast milk is dynamic and changes as time passes, providing the nutritional requirements for your baby's proper growth and development. Once a baby begins eating solids, the amount of breast milk needed will slowly decline, but breast milk will continue to be the primary source of nutrition for at least the first year of life and solids before a year of age are an opportunity for babies to learn, experiment, and become exposed to different tastes.

You may not ever reach forty ounces per day, in which case you will simply want to continue with the initial schedule until you reach about two or three months post-partum. If you do decide to drop a session earlier than this, you run the risk of affecting your supply down the road. While this is not an absolute, you unfortunately will not know until it is too late. It is best to take advantage of your high prolactin levels while you have them, in the early weeks post-partum.

If your supply does reach a peak volume, or you reach approximately the two to three month mark with a supply volume that is meeting or exceeding your baby's needs, you should be at a point at which you can safely start to drop pumping sessions (unless you have an extremely low supply in which case the two to three month mark is irrelevant and it is best to continue to pump often). Drop sessions slowly—no more than one a month is a good guideline. Of course, the rate at which you drop pumping sessions will also be determined by when you want to wean. In general, the longer you want to pump, the more slowly you should drop sessions. We'll talk more about dropping pumping sessions later in this chapter.

Frequency and Length: The Research

Women who are pumping are often told to continue pumping for five minutes once milk stops flowing, but this advice can be dangerous. Some women mistakenly believe that the slowed flow in between let-downs means they are finished, but most women will have multiple let-downs, as we've discussed. Also, research has shown that breasts are never truly "empty" with about twenty percent of available milk remaining in the breast— and this is regardless of whether a mother is directly breastfeeding or fully expressing.[14]

Information from numerous women who exclusively pump indicates that women pump, on average, about 120 minutes within a twenty-four hour period. There has been little research on the length of time required for exclusively pumping breast milk. For many women, the guideline of 120 minutes in a 24 hour period seems to work very well, and it is important to note that this guideline of 120 minutes will continue to be valid for as long as you pump: every time you drop a pumping session, you will add time to your remaining sessions to ensure you are pumping for approximately 120 minutes every day. There has been some research though that suggests a range of times.

One study, conducted by Dr. Jane Morton, that was specifically looking at using hands-on pumping techniques with mothers of pre-term babies, noted that on average pumping sessions lasted about 20 minutes per session, including hands-on techniques such as compression and massage. She discovered that seven or more sessions in a 24 hour period resulted in higher volumes of breast milk within the first couple of weeks, but this didn't continue to hold true for six weeks post-partum. However, supporting the practices of many exclusively pumping moms, she found that fewer but longer sessions after six weeks continued to provide efficient milk removal and production. In the early weeks, Dr. Morton's research showed an average of 140 minutes per 24 hour period, and in the later weeks (six to eight weeks post-partum) a slight increase of 150 minutes per 24 hour session, but with fewer sessions during that 24-hour period.[15, 16]

An older study that looked at breastfeeding patterns in exclusively breastfed infants calculated the total sucking duration of infants during a 24-hour period and at a variety of ages. The amount of breastfeeding time in a 24-hour period was highest in the first couple of weeks at just a little over two hours (120 minutes), which is consistent with what we know about the initiation of supply and the importance of frequent stimulation. After a couple weeks, the median dropped slightly, to just under two hours per 24-hour period and continued to drop, just a little, until about 16 weeks when it was about 90 minutes per day. It is important to note though that this study was for *breastfed* babies and these times cannot simply be assigned to mothers who are expressing milk, although they can be used as a means for understanding patterns.[17]

Be Persistent

It is natural to worry about whether you are making enough milk for your baby's needs, and sometimes the balance may not be in your favour. Early difficulty with breastfeeding may have started things off slowly and affected the initiation of your milk supply, or perhaps you didn't begin pumping right away. Regardless of the cause, it is important to know that your milk supply can increase over the first two or three months. Just because you are struggling with supply now does not mean that this will always be how it is. Many pumping moms find that their supply continues to increase over the first few weeks, but of course this increase requires good pumping habits. Pumping infrequently or with a poor quality breast pump will almost always result in problems. But hang in there, be positive and persistent, and you'll be giving yourself the best chance to build a milk supply sufficient for your baby's needs.

As was mentioned in chapter four, storage capacity apparently increases over the first four months of lactation and you can use this to your advantage by maintaining a frequent and consistent pumping schedule during this time.[18] Other research has shown it possible to increase milk production over the first eight weeks with the addition of hands-on pumping techniques.[19] So while anecdotal evidence suggests to us that increases can happen over the early weeks, research also suggests this possibility. If you are struggling in the early weeks to increase your supply to a volume to meet your baby's needs, this should hearten you. Persistence and patience are virtues, and as moms we often have to exhibit a great deal of patience and persistence. Perhaps this is simply your training ground!

Exclusively Pumping after Breastfeeding

If you have established your supply breastfeeding, the switch to exclusively pumping will require a similar schedule to the one outlined above regardless of how long you were breastfeeding. You will start pumping using 120 minutes per day of pumping as a guideline. There are a few reasons for this:

- Your body will respond to a pump differently than it responded to your baby. You will need to "retrain" your body. You may find that your milk ejection reflex is not as reliable as with your baby and, therefore, it will take longer to remove milk with a pump. The milk ejection reflex is, at least to some extent, a conditioned response, so this frequent pumping schedule will help condition your body to release milk for the pump.
- Your baby may be better at emptying your breasts than a pump will be. Therefore, while your baby may maintain your supply only feeding five times a day, you may not find this the case with a pump, and you will need to pump more frequently than if you were breastfeeding.
- Since it can be more difficult to increase your supply later on when you are exclusively pumping, you will want to increase your supply now in order to allow yourself the ability to drop pump sessions later with a bit of a cushion in case of supply dips.

When making the switch from breastfeeding to exclusively pumping, pump every two to three hours during the day and at least once between 1 a.m. and 5 a.m. Aim for at least six to eight sessions within a twenty-four hour period. The lower your supply and the younger your baby, the more often you will want to pump. Ensure you are pumping approximately 120 minutes a day. Remember though that guidelines need to be personalized. Some women will need to pump more than this and a very few can get away with pumping less. This, however, gives you a good place to start.

My recommendation is to continue to pump at this schedule until your supply exceeds the maximum daily intake that your baby will require (approximately 960 milliliters or thirty-two ounces). If you do produce a high volume, you may attempt to drop a pumping session, but if you are not expressing a high volume, maintain this schedule as long as you can or until you reach at least two to three months post-partum. Remember that for the first month or so post-partum you have higher levels of prolactin assisting you with milk production. Use this to your advantage and establish as strong a supply as you can within this time period.

Individual Considerations

Women will empty their breasts at different rates. Some women have a stronger MER than others. Keep in mind that everyone is different and some women will need to pump longer and some women will find they can maintain a supply pumping less. Also, different pumps will affect the length of time needed to remove milk from the breast; some will be more effective than others. Take the time recommendations offered here as a guideline, and do alter them for your individual situation if need be.

We've already established that the MER is not continuous. Oxytocin, which initiates the MER, is not continuously present but is released in waves. Therefore, just because your milk flow stops does not mean that you have emptied your breasts suffi-ciently. If you continue to breastfeed or pump, you will in most cases experience another let-down. In fact, as we've previously discussed, the common belief that you can empty your breasts is a misconception. Milk is continually produced, making it impossible to completely empty your breasts. Therefore, the often heard advice to pump until your milk stops flowing is not necessarily good advice when it comes to maintaining a strong supply. Keeping track of time, maintaining accurate records, and adding time to your pumping sessions as you drop sessions—all with the aim of consistently achieving at least 120 minutes of pumping each day—is a far better strategy.

In addition, you'll remember that in a previous chapter we discussed the idea that women have different storage capacities and that this will affect milk production. Keep this in mind when determining your pumping schedule. There is no easy way to determine your storage capacity, but it's always a good idea to be cautious initially and to make small changes. Women with larger storage capacities tend to be those who pump large volumes of milk first thing in the morning. These women also will often not see any supply decrease when dropping pumping sessions, and in fact may experience an increase.

Maintaining Your Supply

The key to maintaining your supply for the long term is to create an environment that will allow for optimal milk production, and additionally to remove milk from your breasts. It is that simple. What is not simple, however, is controlling all the variables that can affect your supply, having the stamina to continue a rigorous pumping schedule, and continuing to spend time with your pump instead of your baby. Regardless, the key to maintaining a strong supply is to ensure the milk in your breasts is removed regularly allowing the feedback loop to signal that more milk is to be produced. An excellent breast pump is an absolute necessity, but beyond the pump, there are a number of things you can do to both build a strong supply and maintain it. If your supply declines after a few weeks or months, it is sometimes possible to increase it, but not always.

It is best not to lose your supply in the first place! Be sure to do the following:

- Maintain a good pumping schedule. After taking care of your baby, allow pumping sessions to take priority in your day. There is no quick fix for a haphazard schedule. Remember, you want to aim for around 120 minutes a day. While you do not need to pump at exactly the same time every day, you should aim for the same number of sessions every day and try not to go any longer than six hours between pumping sessions. In fact, in the early days and weeks, I would recommend not going longer than four hours through the day, and to only do this if absolutely necessary.
- Do not drop pumping sessions too early. It is very tempting to drop sessions as quickly as possible, but you don't know how this will affect you down the road. Remember that early on, it is frequency and stimulation that will establish your supply and affect your ability to pump long term. Do not be hasty. The extra effort in the early days will pay off in the long run.
- Reduce the stress in your life when possible — yes, I know you're a new parent and stress is a given, but try to make a place for relaxation and stress reduction — maybe a long shower by yourself or a relaxing walk with your baby. Stress can quickly reduce your milk supply. Relax your expectations and accept help when it's offered.

Share your stress with your friends and partner; let them help shoulder the load.

- Eat well. Caloric and carbohydrate intake are important to milk production. Now is not the time to try to lose extra baby weight (although you might find that just like with breastfeeding, exclusively pumping will help you lose that weight). Be sure you are eating a healthy variety of food and eating enough food. While you do not need to eat a great deal more when lactating than you normally would, you do need to ensure a consistent level of nourishment.

- Drink enough water. The key here is not to become dehydrated. You do not need to drink excessive amounts of water. In fact, some information suggests too much water can have a negative impact on your supply. Drink the recommended 8-10 glasses of water each day, or better yet, drink to thirst, and try to avoid coffees and sodas—which can actually dehydrate you.

- Avoid the use of hormonal birth control containing estrogen. The use of a progestin-only oral contraceptive is preferred if you wish to take birth control pills; however, wait until your supply is well established before starting them. Always monitor your supply closely if you do start any new medication (either prescription or over-the-counter) in case it has a negative impact on your supply.

- Avoid the use of antihistamines. While there is no conclusive verification showing that antihistamines have a negative impact on milk supply, there has been anecdotal evidence suggesting that this can result, and they are often suggested as an aid to rapid weaning. Antihistamines do pass into breast milk, so it is probably best to avoid them for this reason alone.

- Carefully research any medication or herbal supplement before taking it to find out both its effects on lactation and whether it is passed on to the baby through your milk. Motherisk, operated by The Hospital for Sick Children in Toronto, is an excellent resource. They offer extensive information on pregnancy and drug use; breastfeeding and drug use; prescription and over-the-counter medications; and tobacco, alcohol, and illegal drugs. Dr. Thomas Hales' book *Medication and Mother's Milk* is an excellent resource as well, dedicated specifically to breast milk and medications.[20]

- Use an excellent quality double electric hospital-grade breast pump if at all possible. There is no more significant factor in establishing and maintaining a strong supply when pumping than using the best possible breast pump. If you are not finding success, consider trying a different pump for a trial period to see if it makes a difference.

- For specific information on increasing your milk supply—or decreasing it—see Chapter 7, "The Ups and Downs of Pumping: Increasing and Decreasing Supply".

Keeping Records

Type A personalities will love the opportunity to chart and graph and keep extensive records of daily pumping sessions and milk volumes, but everyone will benefit from keeping some type of daily pumping record. A basic notebook can be used simply to jot down the time of your session, perhaps the length, and the amount of milk expressed. Daily totals can quickly be added up and referred back to when required. Some people like to be more formal in their record keeping and may want to use a simple spreadsheet or prepared log sheet. With the popularity of apps for smart phones and tablets, another option is to use an app created for breastfeeding or pumping moms. Many will track pumping sessions and milk storage in addition to tracking baby's wet and dirty diapers, feedings, and many other things. Milk Maid is one such app that is created specifically for pumping moms. It tracks pumping sessions, volumes, stored milk—it even will notify you when milk you have stored is getting close to the maximum recommended storage time. Baby Connect and ifeed are two other apps that have functions for expressed breast milk as well as other tracking features related to general baby care.

Keeping at least basic records will allow you to track supply increases or decreases, note patterns in your supply, remind you of when you have pumped, and can help to track milk you have stored. You can also include information on your baby's intake, which can be of benefit when determining how much milk you need to thaw or how long your current stash might last.

Dropping Pumping Sessions

One of the first questions new mothers will ask when they start to exclusively pump is "When can I drop a pumping session?" While there is no one right answer, it is best not to rush. Remember that it is the first few weeks post-partum that are crucial to establishing a strong milk supply. We know that dropping pumping sessions too quickly can limit the number of prolactin receptors laid down in the breasts. And by dropping sessions too quickly in the first few weeks, you are not taking advantage of the naturally high prolactin levels in your body. For these reasons, as previously discussed, it is best to wait until around two or three months post-partum—or until you have established a strong supply—to drop pumping sessions. Prolactin levels don't suddenly decrease and lactation doesn't magically change from endocrine to autocrine control overnight. It is a gradual process. Prolactin levels have usually returned to close to pre-pregnancy levels by about four weeks post-partum, but waiting an additional four to eight weeks—if you are struggling to build supply—is a good idea. Many women do find that their supply will continue to increase over the first two to three months post-partum with good pumping habits.

Yet some women do choose to drop pumping sessions earlier than this. It is highly individual as to when it is advisable, or perhaps simply necessary, to drop a session for the sake of a person's sanity. Keep in mind your long-term goals and the current daily volume that you are pumping. There is no guarantee what dropping a session will do to your supply. You will have to judge it based on your knowledge of lactation, your supply, and your ability to continue pumping.

The most common reason a woman gives for dropping a pumping session is the need to regain time in her life, to take back some of the time pumping has taken away. This time might be used to sleep, to spend with family, to care for the baby, or a number of other things, but time is what pumping can take away from you and is what most women want to regain. I firmly believe that women know when they need to drop a session. You will just get to a point where it has to be done to maintain balance. Trust your instincts and be comfortable in your decision before you drop the pumping session. Understand that it may negatively affect your supply, and if it does, there is a possibility that you will not be able to regain lost volume—at least not without some considerable effort.

While some women will see an increase in supply when they drop a pumping session, others will see a decrease. This has a lot to do with a woman's storage capacity. If a woman has a large capacity, she often sees an increase in supply simply because she has a longer period of time to produce milk and the capacity to store it—remember the breast is continually producing milk. However, those women with a smaller storage capacity will have to pump more often to achieve the same volumes. Once you understand whether you have a large or small storage capacity, you will be better able to gauge how quickly you can drop sessions and be able to know how few pumping sessions you can do per day without starting to lose your supply.

When dropping a pumping session you have three options:

1. You can drop an actual session and leave the remaining sessions at their usual times. For example if you usually pump at 7a.m., 10 a.m., 1 p.m., 4p.m., 7p.m., 10p.m., and 2 a.m., you may want to drop the 10 a.m. pumping session. Simply dropping the session will allow you a longer stretch of time in the day without having to pump. You may find, however, that you get quite engorged having such a long period between sessions. You may want to pump a little earlier and reduce the length of time between sessions slightly to accommodate your discomfort. Do not allow yourself to get extremely engorged to the point of discomfort or pain. This will only lead to blocked ducts or mastitis. If you are prone to blocks or mastitis, you may be best off dropping sessions by the next method.

2. The second way to drop a pumping session is simply to lengthen the amount of time between all

your remaining sessions. For example, if you had been pumping every three hours, extend this to every four hours. You may still need to pump once or twice after only three hours to fit in all your sessions. An example of this new schedule might be 7 a.m., 11 a.m., 3 p.m., 6 p.m., 10 p.m., and 2 a.m.

3. The third option is not to worry about how long you wait between pumping sessions but instead to pump where and when you can. It is the number of pumping sessions per day as well as the total pumping time throughout the day that is most important. Aim for approximately 120 minutes per day of pumping. Most women find that their volume remains consistent regardless of how long they may go between pumping sessions. If you are trying to pump five times a day, it will make little difference if you pump at 6 a.m., 11 a.m., 4 p.m., 10 p.m., and 3 a.m., or pump at 6 a.m., 9 a.m., 1 p.m., 3 p.m., 9 p.m., and 2 a.m. Both schedules should provide you with the same volumes.

The following are important guidelines to keep in mind when dropping pumping sessions:

- It is best not to go any more than four hours between sessions in the early weeks, and six hours between sessions after a few months of exclusively pumping—and I don't recommend doing this regularly. Remember, the longer milk stays in the breast, the slower production becomes. This is obviously going to be disregarded if you drop down to three pumping sessions a day.

- Do not drop the night session before you reach approximately three months post-partum. You should be pumping at least once between 1 a.m. and 5 a.m. Your prolactin levels are at their highest at night. Take advantage of them. Pumping at night also can free up a bit of extra time throughout the day. While everyone likes their sleep, it may be an option to hold on to this night-time session a bit longer.
- Go slowly when dropping pumping sessions. Consider your long-term goals (the longer you plan to pump, the more slowly you will want to drop sessions). Allow yourself enough time to recognize any negative trends in your supply before you think about dropping another session. A good general guideline is not to drop any more than one session per month (unless, of course, you want to wean).

Chapter 6

The Next Step—Pumping Long Term

I n the last chapter we looked at the basics of establishing your supply and setting up a pumping schedule that will help you maintain your milk supply long term. In this chapter we'll discuss some issues that may come up when exclusively pumping for a longer period and things to consider as you proceed. After the fog of new motherhood has lifted, the excitement of a new baby begins to fade, and things begin to rebalance themselves and "real" life begins to creep back in, the rigors of exclusively pumping can sometimes begin to wear on you. There is no question that exclusively pumping can sometimes be exhausting, but it is also incredibly fulfilling. You are giving your baby something that only you can give and providing the necessary nutrition and building blocks to ensure your baby's optimal development. When you have moments of frustration or exhaustion, remind yourself of the incredible job you are doing and keep your focus on the reasons why you set off on this journey. In this chapter, we will discuss goal setting, creating balance, and keeping things in perspective.

Goal Setting

Many women who exclusively pump past the first couple of months are surprised that they end up exclusively pumping longer than they had perhaps even planned to breastfeed. Once you are able to drop pumping sessions to a less frequent basis, everything becomes more routine and the prospect of continuing less daunting and more achievable. Goal setting is one strategy that can help you continue to pump, even on the days that you feel like quitting.

Setting small, achievable goals and working towards them will allow you to focus on small accomplishments rather than the big challenge. When we start out on a journey, it often seems like a mountain we have to climb, but by focusing on a single step at a time you will get further than you ever imagined. When you start pumping, your goal might be to pump for one month or two months. When you reach that goal, set a new goal. Keep your sights on your goal date, and manage day-by-day and even pump-by-pump if necessary. When you meet your goal you can then reassess it:

- Do you want to continue pumping?
- How is your supply?
- Do you feel you will be able—both physically and mentally—to continue?
- Do you have your family's support?

The answers to these questions will play into your decision to either continue or wean. If you decide to continue, set a new goal and go for it! If you decide to wean, review how to wean in chapter thirteen and take it slow. Depending on how much breast milk you are currently pumping, you should allow yourself between two and four weeks to wean comfortably.

If your supply is not meeting your baby's needs and you are thinking about weaning, you may want, as an alternative, to consider supplementing with formula to make up the short-fall. Any amount of breast milk is beneficial to your child, and breast milk is still far superior to formula. While your baby may not receive 100% breast milk, she does receive 100% of the benefits of your milk. You will need to decide what is best for your baby, but realize that pumping does not have to be an all or nothing proposition if your supply is on the lower end of the scale.

Often, once women meet their long-term goal, they pump on a day-to-day basis, meaning that they take every day pumping as a bonus for their baby. My long-term goal was eight months, when my son would be six months adjusted in age. After reaching this point, I felt very little stress about pumping, knowing that mentally I would be comfortable weaning when I felt ready.

The first few months of exclusively pumping are tiring and demanding but eventually you will hit your stride and things will seem to go more smoothly. Maybe it's that you simply get used to your new schedule and the expectations of your new life as a mother, or maybe it does really get easier. Either way, know that you are not alone and that the emotions you feel at any given time have been felt—and are being felt right now—by others. Becoming a mother can be challenging, regardless of how you're feeding your baby. Some of the stress and emotions you feel in the first weeks and months after your baby is born are just part of this transition process as you ease into your new role and as your hormones try to find some semblance of balance; not everything you experience will necessarily be related to exclusively pumping. When you are struggling, reach out and connect with others who can support you—and sometimes even commiserate with you.

Creating a Balance

For many women, it is easy to become consumed with pumping. Everything, it seems, becomes focused on providing breast milk for your baby. Often this is because mothers feel a sense of loss—often expressed as guilt—about not being able to breastfeed and are determined to make pumping work. This focus, however, can create an imbalance in your life and cause problems within your marriage, with your health, or your overall well-being. It is very important to attempt to look at the larger picture—which admittedly can be difficult—and take active steps to create balance in your life and home:

- Speak openly with your spouse. Explain the importance of feeding breast milk—both the physical and emotional benefits to you and your baby. Enlist his support and understanding. Accept his help. Listen to his concerns. Sometimes a husband's suggestions to wean early are due to concern for you and your health and well-being. Suggest concrete ways that he can support you such as taking the baby for an afternoon while you catch up on rest or making dinner once in a while—or even massaging your feet while you pump.

- Let go of assumptions and expectations. Accept things as they are. Take things as they come. Be willing to bend. Things rarely work out as we expect. You may have expected to breastfeed. You may have expected to have everything in your household under control. Things change. Don't worry about how you thought things were going to be. Focus instead on what you do have and the situation you are now in. Live in the moment and be willing to roll with it.

- Find someone with whom to share your feelings and concerns. Talk it out! Pumping can be very isolating since it may confine you to your home, especially early on. Get support—a friend, an online discussion board, a doctor, a lactation consultant, your mother—anyone who you trust and who is interested in listening, understanding, and supporting.[1]
- Think through worst-case scenarios. What is the worst thing that would happen if you quit pumping? Or lost your supply? Or had to start supplementing with formula? This will either spur you on or give you permission to relax a little and recognize that the alternative isn't so bad.
- If you are running on empty, consider dropping a pumping session. The reason most women give for dropping a session is the need to regain some time to do other things through the day: to sleep more, or to have more time with the baby, other children, or their spouse.

Don't allow pumping to affect your health, your relationship with your baby, or your relationship with your spouse. Keep things in balance. I know this is easier said than done. I get that, and I've been there, but your health and well-being are paramount to the health and well-being of your family.

Look At the Big Picture

When discussing volumes, it is important to step back and get a look at the big picture. While exclusively pumping is done to provide the very best for your baby, it is important not to forget about another important thing a baby needs—a loving mother who is able to respond to her baby's needs.

Work to maintain a balance between establishing and maintaining your supply and maintaining a life that allows you to forge a strong, loving bond with your baby. If you feel like you can't continue as you are, try dropping a pumping session and see what happens. As women we like to put others first, and while it's important that we take care of our family, we are no good to our family if we don't also take care of ourselves.

As well, do not make a rash decision to drop a pump. Ensure you are not making the decision out of frustration, anger, or fatigue. Never drop a pump or decide to wean on a bad day. Often it is best to wait a few days after deciding to drop a session before you actually cut it out of your schedule. Set yourself a goal date when you plan on dropping the session. Once you get to that date, if you still feel it is time to do it and you need to do it, then go ahead and drop it. Do it to maintain a balance in your health, your relationships, and your life.

Every woman who exclusively pumps has days where she does not think she can continue. You won't be the first and you won't be the last. These days are the time to reach out to your support group. Look at the larger picture. Think about why you are doing what you are doing. Weigh the pros and cons. Understand what your options are and how they might affect your long-term goal. Be honest with yourself about your emotions and strive to maintain a balance. Some days you might have to take one pump at a time; throw that long-term goal out the window for the day. Chances are, tomorrow things will look better. But if they don't, it's okay to do what you need to do. Trust yourself and know that you have a lot more determination and strength now that you are a mother. If you want to do it, you'll find a way.

You're Feeding Your Baby, Not the Freezer

Often, women who are exclusively pumping become focused on freezing as much milk as possible. Seeing frozen breast milk in the freezer is tangible proof of your hard work and provides a safety net in case of a supply disaster. A complete change in mindset occurred for me after approximately five months of pumping when someone on the exclusively pumping discussion board at iVillage reminded me that I was pumping to feed my baby, not my freezer.

Up to this point, I was producing far more than my son required. His having been nine weeks premature, I had a very large head start on him in terms of my supply compared to his intake. Within two months, my small apartment-sized freezer was overflowing. I was constantly stressing about where to put the large amount of breast milk I was pumping every day. I was planning to begin rotating my freezer stash: starting to feed frozen breast milk and freezing my fresh milk. But I knew that fresh milk was the best for my baby. After all, why was I going through all the trials of pumping if not to feed my son the best possible?

It was this response to my post on the message board asking for advice about my growing freezer stash, limited freezer space, and the desire to feed my son the best possible, that reminded me that I was doing all this to feed my baby, not my freezer. This comment helped me to regain a balance, gain perspective on my situation, and perhaps made it possible for me to pump for another seven months. From that moment on, I fed my son exclusively fresh milk and culled my freezer stash when necessary to allow me to freeze more fresh milk. I was comfortable knowing that my son was getting the best expressed breast milk possible for as long as I chose to pump—and I knew that I would still have enough frozen milk to feed my son for a couple months after I weaned.

Low Volume

If you are not able to express enough milk to meet your baby's needs, then the discussion of freezing milk and dealing with the large volumes produced may leave you feeling a little disappointed, upset, or frustrated. Do not despair. As has been said previously, any amount of breast milk is beneficial and even though your baby may not be receiving 100% breast milk, he is receiving 100% of the benefit from your breast milk. Many women who do not pump enough for their babies choose to supplement with formula instead of weaning. Some will seek out donor sources of milk. This is a decision that you will have to make.

If you have tried everything and still are not producing the volume your baby requires, then you will perhaps simply have to accept it. I know, that's not the most supportive attitude, is it? But in all honesty, you are giving your best to your child, and there is no fault or guilt in that. There is nothing to be ashamed of—and everything to feel proud of! You have the courage and determination to continue pumping! You are showing true dedication to your baby by providing her with breast milk, and the amount you pump truly has no bearing on the value of the gift you are giving her.

Chapter 7

The Ups and Downs of Pumping: Increasing and Decreasing Supply

One of the most common questions pumping moms ask is "How can I increase my supply?" Ideally, with good pumping (or breastfeeding) practices from the start, you will never need to ask this question. But the fact is that many women—for a multitude of reasons—experience low milk supply at some point. And while a low supply can cause concern and challenges, an exceedingly large supply can also bring its own set of problems. While a woman with a large supply may not need to worry about having enough milk for her baby, she may be more inclined to suffer from engorgement, blocked ducts, or mastitis. In this chapter, we'll look at both ends of the supply spectrum and discuss strategies for boosting and reducing your supply.

Low Milk Supply

The basics of lactation clearly indicate that a mother's milk supply is determined by supply and demand. So it would seem simple to solve a low supply—simply increase the demand. This, in its simplest form, is the best advice you can get. And increasing the demand by adding pumping sessions is the first thing you should do if you need to boost your supply. Generally speaking, by increasing the frequency of pumping and thereby increasing demand, your milk supply should increase. Likewise, we know that milk left sitting in the breast will start to slow milk production, so ensuring as much milk as possible is removed as frequently as possible should help to maintain and increase production. It would seem simple, right? But the reasons for low milk supply can sometimes be challenging to pinpoint, and when you consider that nature didn't intend for a pump to be the source of milk removal and stimulation, there is a new layer of complexity added to the mix.

The best way to address a low milk supply is to avoid it in the first place. Accurate information, a frequent pumping schedule, full milk removal, an excellent quality double-electric pump: all these things will help you establish a strong supply from the start. But if complicating factors are involved—or you didn't have access to good information when you first started exclusively pumping and are now struggling with supply—you need to work with what you've got, try to identify anything that is hindering your supply, and move forward implementing strategies to help you boost it.

Reasons for Low Milk Supply and Strategies to Boost It

The reasons for a low milk supply can sometimes be rather elusive. There are, however, some common causes to consider. If you have not been able to initiate a sufficient supply, or your supply has decreased, consider the following possible reasons for a low supply or decreased supply and strategies and techniques for boosting it:

- Could you possibly have a blocked duct or mastitis? Both can dramatically reduce your supply. See the chapter entitled "Overcoming Challenges" for symptoms and treatments.

- Are you getting enough sleep? Although sleep and babies do not always go together, it is important that you are as rested as possible. Can someone else take care of the baby for awhile so you can rest? Could you hire a babysitter so you can get some shut-eye?

- Is your pump working as it should? Take your pump apart and check for any tears in the membranes or valves, holes in the tubing, or blockages. Listen to the pump's motor: does it sound like it is working well? Put the flange up to your cheek and turn the pump on. Does it create suction? If you are concerned your low supply may be a result of your pump, call the pump manufacturer or find a local rental depot or lactation consultant who can test the pump's suction level to ensure it is working optimally.

- Have you recently started taking any type of medication: prescription or non-prescription? Check to see if this medication could possibly reduce your milk supply. While you may have asked if it was safe for your baby, your doctor might have overlooked the effects on lactation. Dr. Thomas Hale's book *Medication and Mother's Milk* is an excellent resource providing information on the impact of medications on mother's milk. Your pharmacist is another good source of information regarding medications and lactation. Common culprits include hormonal birth control

(including IUDs that have a hormone component) and cold medications.

- Are you eating enough and eating well? While
  lactation will happen regardless of what you eat,
  poor diet can affect you in numerous other ways.
  It can cause you to get run-down leading to illness; it can affect your ability to handle stress;
  and it can affect your overall sense of well-being.
  Your milk supply may decrease if you are not
  taking in enough calories; however, it is certain
  that the fat content of your milk will be adversely
  affected. If your milk has a low fat content, your
  baby will need more milk to meet her caloric
  needs. If your supply is also reduced, this may
  create a problem. Sufficient calories and carbohydrates are a definite must.

- Are you dehydrated? While super-hydrating can
  bring its own set of problems, you do need to ensure you are drinking to thirst and staying well
  hydrated. It is not necessary, however, to drink
  excessive amounts of water. Establish a routine
  of drinking a glass of water whenever you sit
  down to pump and you should be fine.

- Have you considered oatmeal? Try eating oatmeal daily. Many women give anecdotal support
  to the value of oatmeal to increase their milk
  supply. Oatmeal in any form will work—even
  oatmeal cookies! Consider starting your day with
  a bowl of hot oatmeal. Some mothers report similar effects from drinking non-alcoholic beer,
  which may also increase the antioxidant levels of
  breast milk.[1] The barley in beer can potentially

increase prolactin; however there is no clear evidence for this.[2]

- Are herbal galactogogues part of your daily routine? Herbal supplements such as fenugreek, goat's rue, anise, basil, blessed thistle, fennel seeds, and marshmallow or a combination of herbs found in ready-made supplements, such as Mother's Milk Tea, have traditionally been used to help women increase their milk supply.[3] Fenugreek is the most common herbal supplement for increasing supply. It smells like maple syrup, and if you take enough of it, you too will smell like maple syrup. Fenugreek has been associated with gassiness and stomach irritability in both mother and baby, so be watchful for those symptoms. If your baby is premature and in the hospital, it is best to check with the neonatologist before starting any supplements that might pass through your milk to your baby. Women who are allergic to ragweed, peanuts, chickpeas, soybeans, and green peas should be cautious as they may also react to fenugreek. Interactions are also possible for hypoglycemics (including insulin), and those taking aspirin, heparin, warfarin, feverfew, primrose, and other herbals.[4] As is always the case, consultation with a medical professional, herbalist, or naturopath is recommended.
- Are you dealing with the stress in your life? Having a new baby brings with it a certain amount of stress, and exclusively pumping — especially if it was not what you intended on doing — can also add a certain amount of stress. But reducing the

stress in your life as much as possible will assist your efforts to increase and maintain your supply. Many women find that when they are highly stressed they have a marked decrease in their daily milk volume. Avoid it when you can; deal with it in healthy ways when you can't. Try exercising, find a support group either in your community or online, journal daily to release emotions, pray, and lean on those around you who care about you. Really, it's all about self-care and it's a great lesson to learn early as many moms forget about the need to care for themselves. Often stress will affect supply due to the effect of stress and tension on the milk ejection response. Since oxytocin is a "shy" hormone that doesn't like to show itself if there is fear or stress, learning relaxation techniques can help with oxytocin release.

- Are you in pain? As with stress, pain can reduce oxytocin release and in turn reduce let-down. Resolving the pain will help improve oxytocin release. See chapter 12 for information on the common causes of pain when pumping.

- Have you recently started your period? Hormones can play havoc with your milk supply. While your supply will usually improve after your period ends, it might not always pick back up to its former volume. If you find your period returns while still pumping and your supply decreases just prior to and during your period, try taking calcium and magnesium supplements. The suggested dosage is between 500 mg calcium and 250 mg magnesium to 1500 mg calcium and

750 mg magnesium.[5] It is best to start taking the supplements about one week prior to the beginning of your period and continue taking it throughout.

- Have you started taking hormonal birth control? Just as the hormone fluctuations of your monthly cycle can affect lactation, the hormones contained within hormonal contraceptives can also reduce milk supply. It is always a good idea to delay any type of hormonal birth control until your milk supply is well established, and even then it is best to use a progestin-only form. While opinions on hormonal birth control and its potential impact on milk supply vary, there have been numerous anecdotal reports of milk supply dropping as a result of starting hormonal contraception. If you've started it and your supply has diminished, stop taking it and increase your pumping frequency to see if your supply rebounds. If you are considering birth control, check out your options and consider a non-hormonal form, especially if your milk supply is on the lower end of the spectrum or you are still in the first few months post-partum.

- Do you have a medical condition or lifestyle that may cause low milk supply? Common conditions that could affect supply include pregnancy, certain medications, glandular insufficiency (hypoplasia), previous breast surgery, diabetes, polycystic ovarian syndrome (PCOS), hypothyroidism, retained placenta, theca lutein cyst, post-partum hemorrhage, smoking, and heavy alcohol use.[6]

Be sure to also see chapter 5 for the tips and techniques that will help you build and maintain your milk supply when exclusively pumping. And remember, above all else, frequency and consistency are most important.

Prescription Medications

Pharmaceutical galactogogues (medications—and herbs—that can assist with lactation initiation or increasing production) are available and are a consideration for some women. All medications currently used as galactogogues work as dopamine antagonists, which will increase prolactin levels.[7] A dopamine antagonist blocks the dopamine receptors. As was mentioned in the chapter on lactation and breast milk composition, dopamine has an inverse relationship with prolactin. As dopamine increases, prolactin decreases. While there is no evidence that increased prolactin levels result in increased milk volume,[8] dopamine antagonists are sometimes used to assist women with milk production.

Domperidone and metoclopramide are the prescription drugs frequently prescribed to increase milk supply. Both are most effective in mothers of premature babies who are having difficulty establishing a supply, in the early days and weeks of lactation, or for mothers who experience a drop in supply, often related to the use of birth control pills.[9] These drugs should only be considered when other options have been exhausted. While both metoclopramide and domperidone increase the levels of prolactin in the lactating mother, they will not make up for poor pumping habits or allow you to pump less often.

The Academy of Breastfeeding Medicine stresses that there are only a few well-done studies looking into the effectiveness of these medications. They encourage medical professionals and mothers to carefully weigh the potential side-effects against the lack of evidence.[10] In some cases the potential risks will outweigh the potential benefits, but not in every situation. Make a decision based on research and consultation with a doctor.

Depression is a reported side-effect of metoclopramide (with the brand names of Reglan or Maxeran). Other possible side-effects include dizziness, nausea, sweating, anxiety, sedation, restlessness, and gastric cramping.[11, 12] Reglan has been involved in lawsuits resulting from the more serious side-effects. One such serious side-effect is called Tardive Dyskinesia, which is a condition that seriously affects movement. If taking metoclopramide, you should start to see an increase in your supply within two or three days.

Because metoclopramide crosses the blood-brain barrier and brings with it a real risk of depression, domperidone is often considered the preferred choice of prescription medications for increasing milk supply. Depression is not a side-effect associated with domperidone. It does bring with it the possibility of dry mouth, abdominal cramping, and headaches, which often go away when the dosage is reduced.[13, 14]

It is important to note that domperidone is not approved in any country for use by breastfeeding mothers in order to increase milk production. In most cases, this does not preclude you from using it in this way. However, the Food and Drug Administration (FDA) in the United States of America did issue a release in June of 2004 warning against women using domperidone to increase their milk supply. They highlight that the distribution or importation of the drug is illegal in the U.S.A. While you cannot buy domperidone ready made in the U.S.A., you can sometimes have it compounded at a compounding pharmacy with a doctor's prescription. In March 2012, Health Canada released a similar warning about the use of domperidone for off-label uses; however in Canada—and in other countries—you are able to get domperidone with a prescription. It is important to note, however, that the FDA's initial warning was in response to the possible cardiac side-effects of domperidone administered intravenously to sick patients, and not domperidone given orally to breastfeeding women. These warnings have created a lot of controversy in the lactation community.

Still, if you are considering the use of either domperidone or metoclopramide, you need to seek the advice of a doctor who is knowledgeable about breastfeeding and the use of these drugs to increase breast milk supply. Both drugs have the potential for negative drug interactions and so a doctor should be consulted to review your health history before starting either domperidone or metoclopramide.

Power Pumping and Cluster Pumping

If you need to increase your supply, there are a couple of pumping techniques you can try: power pumping and cluster pumping. Power pumping requires frequent pumping through-out the day. You should pump at least every two hours around the clock for at least two days, but can pump as often as every hour or hour and a half. Power pumping is essentially trying to mimic a growth spurt by removing as much milk as possible and signaling your body to make more milk to meet the demand. The best way to increase your supply is to remove more milk from your breasts more frequently and increase the amount of stimulation to the breasts, nipples, and areolas.

Some women who power pump will spend a weekend com-mitted to the process. They will enlist the help of family or friends to care for the baby so that they can focus on pumping frequently. Having multiple sets of flanges and lots of collection bottles, so you do not need to wash and sterilize after each pumping session, can also assist in making it through the rigorous power pumping schedule.

Cluster pumping is a variation on power pumping. In this case you will be pumping frequently, as with power pumping.

However, you will pump for shorter periods. For example, you will pump every half hour for ten minutes at a time. Do this for two to four hours at a time. The benefit to cluster pumping is that you can do it for only a portion of the day and then repeat it every few days. You will need to stay close to your pump while cluster pumping, but it will not require the multiple day commitment of power pumping.

Pumps and Technique

Really, when it comes down to it, expressing breast milk has been made quite easy with the development of modern breast pumps. Yet, as will be discussed in the upcoming chapter, "Pumps and Kits, Oh My!", not all pumps are created equal. And while the process of expressing breast milk is fairly straightforward, there are some techniques that can be used to make milk expression more effective and efficient. If you are trying to increase your supply, using all of the little tricks and techniques possible can make a difference. Here is a list of points to consider and strategies to implement:

- Whenever possible, use a double-electric pump.
- If you have the financial resources, rent or purchase a hospital-grade pump.
- Consider trying a different type of pump, and preferably a pump by a different manufacturer as pumps are not created equally and work in different ways.
- Use warm compresses on your breasts prior to pumping, or take a warm shower.
- Massage your breasts before you begin to pump. Or start with some hand expression, moving your fingers from the chest wall and rolling towards the areola.

- Lean forward and allow your breasts to hang freely while raking your fingernails gently from the chest wall towards the areola and nipple. Alternatively, you might use a wide comb instead of your fingernails.

- Use breast compressions during your pumping session and massage out any spots that may be hard. As mentioned in an earlier chapter, breast compressions simply require you to hold your breast in a C-hold with the fingers on one side of the breast and thumb on the opposite side. Keep the fingers well back of the areola as pressure in this area may actually stop milk flow. Squeeze firmly but not to the point of discomfort. Hold until you feel the milk release or you need to reposition your hand. Using a hands-free pumping bra can definitely assist you in doing compressions while pumping.

- Be sure to alternate the cycling speed and suction strength during your session. Start with a fairly fast cycling speed and low suction until you begin to let down. Then at this point, switch to a slower cycling speed and higher suction (only as high as you need to remove milk and remain comfortable). Once milk flow slows, you can switch back to the initial setting configuration until you get a second let-down. Most women will get at least two let-downs per session.

A Tasty Option

There are a number of different foods that are anecdotally reported to increase milk supply. As mentioned above, oatmeal and beer are two such food items. Adding lactogenic foods—

foods that help to increase milk production—to your diet can be as simple as adding a bowl of oatmeal to your regular routine, but there are many tasty lactation boosting recipes available online. One of the first such recipes is Noel Trujillo's recipe: Housepoet's Famous Lactation Boosting Oatmeal, Chocolate Chip, and Flaxseed Cookies. While no scientific studies have been done to prove their efficacy, they are absolutely delicious and with the benefits of oatmeal, brewer's yeast, and flax, they certainly can't hurt!

Housepoet's Famous Lactation Boosting Oatmeal, Chocolate Chip, and Flaxseed Cookies

1 cup butter or margarine
1 cup sugar
1 cup brown sugar
4 tablespoons water
2 tablespoons flax meal
2 large eggs
1 teaspoon vanilla
2 cups flour
1 teaspoon baking soda
1 teaspoon salt
3 cups oats, thick cut if you can find them
1 cup chocolate chips
2 tablespoons brewer's yeast

Preheat oven to 375 degrees F. Mix together 2 tablespoons of flaxseed meal and water, and set aside for 3-5 minutes. Cream margarine and sugar. Add eggs one at a time, mix well. Stir flaxseed mixture and add with vanilla to the margarine mix. Beat until blended. Sift together dry ingredients, except oats and chocolate chips. Add to margarine mixture. Stir in oats, then chocolate chips. Scoop or drop onto baking sheet, preferably lined with parchment paper or silpat. The dough is a little crumbly, so it helps to use a scoop. Bake 8-12 minutes, depending on the size of cookies. Makes 6 dozen cookies.[15]

Donor Milk

Formula is usually the go-to option if you need to supplement your own breast milk, but there is another option: donor milk. Donor milk has been used for centuries—likely from the beginning of time—in the form of wet nurses. Today, other options are available and are something you may consider if you find you are not quite able to supply enough milk for your baby. In recent years mother to mother sharing of breast milk has garnered media attention, sometimes in a sensationalistic way, but at the heart of breast milk donation is a desire to help other mothers and give babies the best possible start in life.

There are a number of milk banks throughout North America (and around the world); however, most of the milk from milk banks is used for hospitalized infants and not available for most babies. The Human Milk Banking Association of North America (HMBANA) is a non-profit organization that works to establish milk banks, manage policy, and promote the interests of human milk banking.[16] There are also for-profit milk banks such as Prolacta; although again, milk from this organization is primarily for the use of hospitalized infants and many people have issues with the idea of a for-profit milk bank, believing it should be given for altruistic purposes.

So where can you turn for milk if you'd like to use human donor milk instead of formula? In recent years, organizations such as Eats on Feets and Human Milk 4 Human Babies have been created to help connect moms with milk with moms who need milk.[17] As with anything else, you should investigate carefully and be comfortable with the potential risks. Organizations such as these go a long way to promote normal infant feeding and removing the stigma of breastfeeding and breast milk. They focus on moms helping moms, and that's a great thing!

Oversupply

While it might at first seem like a problem you'd like to have, oversupply can be difficult to deal with. Women with oversupply issues often suffer from recurrent blocked ducts, mastitis, engorgement, and such an abundance of milk that their freezers quickly fill and storage becomes a problem. Oversupply can often cause difficulties for a mother and breastfeeding baby and may be a reason why a mother begins to exclusively pump. However, exclusively pumping may not resolve the issues for the mother and may create further concerns if the breasts are not emptied fully or supply is allowed to increase even further.

It is always good practice to keep records of your pumping sessions and how much milk you are expressing. When you have oversupply, record keeping is very important so you can track your production and take steps to avoid your supply from increasing too much. The normal milk intake for a baby ranges from around 25-35 oz/day. Giving yourself a buffer of several ounces is not a bad idea, as it can give you a cushion for sudden supply drops and allow you to begin storing milk in your freezer in the event that you'd like to wean and continue feeding breast milk. However, milk supply in excess of 45 or 50 oz. is unnecessary—unless you are feeding multiples—and you may want to actively prevent your supply from increasing too far beyond this point.

Women with large milk supplies are usually women who have large storage capacities. Since milk production will slow as the breast fills, women with large storage capacities often find that they can go for an extended period between pumping sessions and their supply is maintained and sometimes will even increase. The problem, however, is that milk that is left sitting in the breast, and breasts that are never fully emptied, can leave a woman prone to blocked ducts and mastitis. So a balance between full milk removal and frequency needs to be found.

Although not as common, oversupply can result from hormonal imbalances and problems with the hypothalamus or pituitary gland. If your supply is continuing to increase despite your efforts to maintain or reduce it, you may want to consider speaking to your doctor or a lactation consultant about checking for potential medical causes of oversupply. Although I wouldn't suggest taking extreme measures on your own, you may want to have a chat with your doctor or lactation consultant about the possible use of medication to reduce supply. Pseudoephedrine can quickly reduce supply (handy to know if you don't want to reduce supply) and estrogen-containing birth control can have a similar effect. To avoid taking too much and reduce your supply to the extreme, it is best to get professional advice on this matter.

For breastfeeding mothers who have oversupply, blocked feeding and full drainage is often used. This means that a mother would offer her baby the same breast for a certain block of time, ensuring that it is fully drained before offering the other breast. For a pumping mom, this technique may not work quite as well since an oversupply when pumping is usually significantly more than oversupply when breastfeeding, and extending the length of time between pumping sessions may simply leave you prone to blocked ducts and mastitis. Instead, by tracking supply and slowly reducing the length of sessions you can begin to reduce the demand. Cut back a couple minutes off of your sessions at a time. Don't make any drastic changes though. It is important to make a plan and see it through. Dropping sessions too quickly, or reducing the length of the sessions too dramatically, may leave you open to blocked ducts and mastitis—and that is definitely something you want to avoid if you can.

Start by reducing the length of your sessions by only a couple minutes. Hold it there until you see what effect that small change has. Once you've reduced your sessions by a few minutes, you can also begin to stretch the time between sessions. Work to remove as much milk as you can during your pumping session, but do not continue to pump if the majority of milk has been removed and your breasts are soft. Continuing to stimulate the breasts once milk has been removed will signal your breasts to increase production, which is not what you want if you have oversupply. The management of your supply will be a fine balance. Continue to reduce the length of sessions, and increase the length of time between sessions, slowly until your supply has been reduced to a volume with which you're happy. Throughout the process, ensure that you are emptying your breasts of milk as much as possible without extending the length of your session. This will require you to use lots of breast compressions during your session.

In addition to the medications mentioned above, there are some herbal supplements that can be taken to reduce supply. Peppermint, sage, and oregano are common herbs that can reduce supply. The sage you season your turkey with is unlikely to have much of an effect, but taking capsules may help. Start with a minimal dose and wait to see what the effect will be. You don't want to obliterate your supply, only reduce it to a manageable level.

Lack of Storage Space

If you are freezing large amounts of breast milk, you may find that your freezer space soon disappears. You might consider buying a larger freezer. A stand-up model is easier to fill and makes it easier to rotate the frozen milk. Another option is to store extra milk in a family member's, friend's, or neighbour's freezer. It might take a bit more in terms of planning and logistics to track the milk and ensure you have enough on hand to meet your needs, but if buying a freezer is not possible and you have a good amount of breast milk you want to freeze, this might be an option. A full freezer works more efficiently and is more cost effective to run; you might want to remind your friends and family of that when you appeal to them for help.

Donate to a Milk Bank

For those women who find themselves with a more-than-ample supply and limited freezer space, the question that eventually arises is "What do I do with all this milk?" In some situations, donating your milk may be the answer. Prematurity, adoption, maternal death, babies with metabolic disorders, allergies and intolerances, and immunological deficiencies are examples of why human breast milk may be required from a donated source.[18]

In Canada, British Columbia, Alberta, and Ontario now have non-profit milk banks connected to the Human Milk Banking Association of North America (HMBANA). In the United States, milk banks are more plentiful. Milk banks are located in California, Texas, North Carolina, Iowa, Michigan, Oregon, Ohio, Massachusetts, Missouri, Indiana, Florida, Mississippi, Delaware, and Colorado. However, due to limited resources, both financial and physical, milk banks may not always be able to accept donations. Contact the closest milk bank to check their donation status, and if they are not accepting at that time, widen your search from there. Some banks will pay for expenses associated with storage and shipping. There are also milk banks in numerous other countries throughout the world. Check to see whether donating to a milk bank is possible where you live. There are also some for-profit milk banks operating; however, consider who is benefiting from your donation. Donating through a non-profit organization ensures no one is profiting from your gift — except for the baby that receives your milk.

Another option is to donate milk directly to another mother. Organizations such as Eats on Feets and Human Milk 4 Human Babies assist in connecting mothers for this purpose.[19]

When donating your milk through a milk bank, your health will be thoroughly checked and blood testing will be required to screen for various illnesses. It is also important that you have not taken any medication or herbal supplements while pumping. There are a few exceptions to this such as insulin or pre-natal vitamins. Check with the milk bank for a list of exceptions. Ineligibility would also arise from other risk factors such as consumption of alcohol, cigarette smoking, being at high risk for HIV due to lifestyle or partner's HIV status or lifestyle, blood transfusion or organ transplant within six months of lactation, as well as certain travel histories.

Selling human milk is illegal in Canada but not in the United States, and other countries have differing laws. However, many moms feel that donating milk is a true act of kindness. By donating your milk, you will be helping another child receive the best possible start to life and you will affect that child into the future.

Chapter 8

Pumps and Kits, Oh My!

One of the most important predictors of successful long-term, exclusive pumping is the pump. In order to build and maintain a strong supply, you must remove the milk from your breasts. That is milk production at its most basic level of supply and demand. A baby that is latching well and removing milk effectively does a great job of building and maintaining supply on their own, but when you use a breast pump it is important to realize that all pumps are not created equal and to choose one that is best suited to the demands of exclusively pumping and your own personal situation.

So Many Options

With so many different breast pumps on the market, it can be difficult to know what will work best, what features are really needed, and what is just hype and marketing. An electric pump that allows you to adjust both the suction level as well as the number of cycles is preferred and will allow you to individualize the pump to meet your own needs. It is important that you use a pump that will allow you to express both breasts at the same time (referred to as double pumping); not only will this save you time, but it can increase your milk volume.[1] Another important consideration is the purpose for which the pump was originally created. There are many good breast pumps on the market; however, many of these were not intended for the extended and frequent use of exclusively pumping. While they might do a satisfactory job for a while, it is possible that the motor may be over-taxed, resulting in decreased performance over time—which in turn will result in decreased supply for you—or they simply may not provide enough stimulation to initiate and maintain a strong supply. Most reputable pump companies recognize the unique needs of exclusively pumping moms and will identify the pumps in their product line that meet or exceed an exclusively pumping mother's needs. Asking other women who are exclusively pumping is also a good way to get recommendations and learn about the benefits of the various types of pumps.

Looking at the operation of the breast pump, it is important that it supplies the right amount of suction and the necessary number of suck and release cycles per minute (cycling). A breastfeeding baby creates between 40 and 60 suck and release cycles per minute and a baby's maximum suction is around 200 to 220 mm Hg (millimeters of Mercury, which is a measure of pressure). While many breast pumps do fall within these ranges, there are a number that do not. Before settling on a pump, find out its specifications. Choose one that will provide the cycles and suction as closely resembling a baby as possible.

In the United States, the Affordable Health Care Act has brought changes to mothers' access to breast pumps. As of January 2013, insurance companies in the U.S.A. are now required to cover the cost of breast pumps; however, there are qualifications and limitations put in place by some companies. Sometimes you'll be required to purchase a specific type of pump and sometimes you'll require a letter from your doctor indicating the breast pump is medically necessary. Check with your insurance company if you live in the United States of America. For Canadians, breast pumps can be claimed as a medical expense on your taxes if you have a doctor's letter. In other countries, check with your own insurance companies and taxation office to see what expenses might be covered.

When choosing a breast pump, the lower cost pumps can be appealing; however, it is important to realize that almost all baby product companies have a breast pump among their product offerings and that many of these pumps are very inefficient and may not even serve a breastfeeding mother very well—let alone an exclusively pumping mother. Often, these pumps are offered simply to complete a product line or to position the company as being "breastfeeding friendly" while the majority of their profits come from bottle feeding and formula feeding supplies. Beware of these pumps if you are exclusively pumping!

Instead, look for a company that focuses primarily on breast pumps and breastfeeding. These companies will continually strive to improve their products and conduct research that will benefit pumping moms. Companies that fit into this description are Medela, Ameda, Hygeia, Limerick, Spectra, and Bailey Medical. However, while these companies focus their efforts to support breastfeeding and breastfeeding mothers, this does not mean that all of their breast pumps will be suitable for an exclusively pumping mother. Do your own research.

Before deciding on a breast pump, learn about your options. Read the rest of this chapter. Go online and search for more information about breast pumps. Chat with other women who are exclusively pumping. Talk to a lactation consultant for her recommendations. Rent a pump and see if it works for you. Most importantly, choose a pump that will be able to withstand the rigors of exclusive pumping.

International Code of Marketing of Breast Milk Substitutes

This might seem to be an odd topic to raise in a chapter about breast pumps, but I do think it is an important one, and one which all parents should be aware of. The International Code of Marketing of Breast Milk Substitutes has been in place since 1981. It was prepared by the World Health Organization (WHO) and adopted by the World Health Assembly. The Code's purpose is to protect infant health by protecting and promoting breastfeeding. It places limits on how breast milk substitutes are marketed and advertised, with the intention of preventing formula and other complementary foods from being marketed in any way that would undermine breastfeeding.[2] In short, the Code is in place to limit commercially motivated interference with breastfeeding that may abbreviate or terminate the mother's breastfeeding option.[3] While breast pumps are not specifically covered by the WHO Code, bottles and bottle nipples are and it is here that companies sometimes break the Code.

Companies that idealize bottle feeding or undermine the importance of breastfeeding are not meeting the Code. Companies that encourage the use of their products in a way that undermines successful breastfeeding (e.g. stating that you should begin pumping soon after your baby is born goes against good breastfeeding practices) are breaking the Code. Is this important to you? I know it is important to me. I want to support companies that are truly supporting mothers, and not placing their end-of-year figures above the health and welfare of babies. Many companies that sell breast pumps have also been accused of not meeting the Code. If you are interested in supporting companies that work hard to sell quality pumps but also follow the Code of Marketing of Breast Milk Substitutes, organizations such as the International Baby Food Action Network (IBFAN)[4] can provide you with a substantial amount of information about the Code and Code breakers. Breast pump companies that are Code compliant include Hygeia, Limerick, and Bailey Medical—unfortunately, a very short list.[5]

Some Supporting Research

Ten years ago as I wrote the first edition of *Exclusively Pumping Breast Milk* the research available on the topic of breast pumps and expressed breast milk was limited. Most of what had been published had been completed with specific focus on the use of breast milk in milk banks. Peter Hartmann, a researcher in Australia, had begun significant work on milk expression and has over the past decade greatly added to our understanding of lactation and milk expression. Yet research in this area is still quite limited and very little relates to long-term exclusive pumping. Some of the current research can perhaps be generalized to exclusively pumping, but more research is definitely needed. Unfortunately, as with everything in life, it seems, you do need to be aware of who is funding the research and how the conclusions benefit those organizations. In the end, the best "research", in my opinion, continues to be the experience of the many women who are exclusively pumping. These women are the ones with the experience and the ones showing that not only is long-term, exclusive pumping possible but showing how best to do it.

Having said that, there have been research studies done that provide important knowledge for exclusively pumping moms. An older study, still relevant today, showed a significant difference in the ability of various breast pumps to produce a strong prolactin response in lactating mothers. The best type of breast pump was found to be an electric pulsatile breast pump.[6] As well, a distinct increase in the production of breast milk has been seen when double pumping, compared to single pumping, was utilized by the pumping mother.[7] More recent research has

141

suggested that combining the use of an electric pump with hands-on pumping (compression and massage) and the use of hand expression to express colostrum in the early days can help to increase milk supply.[8,9] Regardless of the limited amount of research related to exclusively pumping, over the past ten years I have heard from hundreds and hundreds of women who are successfully pumping long term. Their experience proves that it is possible and, with the right information and support, exclusively pumping can be a viable alternative to formula feeding.

Open Vs. Closed Milk Collection Systems

Breast pumps operate on either an open system or a closed system. An open system means that there is no barrier between the milk and the tubing, and therefore the motor, of the pump. In a closed system, there is a barrier in place that prevents any contact between the milk and the tubing and other internal parts of the pump.

All hospital-grade pumps work on a closed system allowing the pump to be used by multiple women without fear of cross-contamination. However, not all personal pumps work on a closed system. If purchasing your own new breast pump, whether the pump has an open or closed system really does not affect you as long as you keep your pump and kit well maintained, although this does mean that you should not loan or give your pump to someone else when you are done with it. Some open system pumps do have the problem of milk entering the tubing and potentially even the motor. If not noticed or cleaned, milk left in the tubing can lead to mold. It is for this reason that open system pumps should be considered single-user pumps as they do run the risk of contaminants entering breast milk. It is strongly recommended that you do not purchase or borrow a previously used open system breast pump.[10, 11] If you choose to use a previously used pump, know the risks.

There are a few companies that do offer personal breast pumps that can be safely used by multiple users. Ameda pumps use what they call a HygieniKit. This kit has a patented silicone diaphragm that prevents milk particles from entering the tubing or motor, thereby protecting subsequent users of the breast pump. Hygeia is another company that offers closed system personal pumps. Hygeia's EnJoye pump has a proprietary filtration system that prevents contaminants from entering the pump. A newer option in the North American market is the Spectra M1 and Spectra 9 breast pumps. All Spectra pumps have a backflow protector to prevent milk from reaching either the tubing or the pump's motor. The Avent Isis IQ Duo is another closed-system pump. For each pump, each woman must use her own collection kit.

Types of Pumps

There are a number of different types of breast pumps on the market and new pumps are always being introduced, while others are discontinued. While the effectiveness of a breast pump is somewhat individual—meaning that some women will respond better to one type of pump and other women do well with another type, given the importance of initiating and maintaining a strong milk supply, I think it is usually best to stay with what is tried and true.

Breast pumps range from inexpensive to very expensive. The less expensive pumps will almost never be appropriate for long-term, exclusive pumping. But this doesn't mean that you need to go out and spend close to a thousand dollars for a hospital-grade breast pump. You do have options, but know your options and fit them to your situation.

Most breast pumps use suction as a means of eliciting let-down and removing milk. This type of pump is most commonly used by exclusively pumping moms and has proved effective for long-term pumping. Pumps in this category include those made by Hygeia, Ameda, Medela, Spectra, and Avent. Other breast pump designs work using gentle compression and stimulation to initiate a let-down and the suctions levels are significantly reduced. Pumps in this category include Simplisse and the Playtex Embrace. A third option is a pump that uses both compression and vacuum. PJ's Comfort by Limerick is a pump that offers both. Research by Dr. M. Woolridge suggests babies use both positive and negative pressure when nursing[12] and the combination of both in a breast pump is an approach that has merit.

Pumps that utilize compression are often reported as being more comfortable, but as with many things relating to exclusively pumping, there has been little research to show that long-term exclusive pumping with this type of pump provides similar and consistent results—however, I haven't seen any research that shows the opposite. One study did compare the use of pumps that use compression with pumps that use suction, and the results showed comparable impacts on lactation. However, you should know that the women participating in the study were exclusively breastfeeding mothers who were returning to work or school, and not women who used the pump to initiate or maintain lactation solely with the pump.[13] It is interesting to note that these two types of pumps appeared to stimulate two different aspects of milk production. The more traditional pump was shown to empty the breast better, while the compression type of pump stimulated the endocrine system to a greater degree and resulted in higher prolactin levels. While higher prolactin is good, I think the better option is to use a traditional style of pump, which has been effectively used by many exclusively pumping mothers on a long-term basis, and also to implement hands-on pumping techniques to increase stimulation to the breast and areola which may in turn help boost prolactin levels. PJ's Comfort pump, which combines both compression and suction, is another option that may indeed benefit prolactin levels and milk removal.

Within each type of pump category, pumps still have further variation. Companies design pumps with unique expression phases, stimulation or let-down phases, and varying patterns of suction and release. Some, like the Bailey Nurture III, require the mother to control the cycling by covering and uncovering a small valve with her finger or thumb repeatedly throughout the pumping session. It is unfortunate that pumps can't be tested for a while in order to find the best one for you, but knowing that they all work just a bit differently is important information to know if the one you are using is simply not working for you. Sometimes switching to a different brand of pump will be helpful in addressing concerns with comfort or effectiveness.

Manual Breast Pumps

Manual pumps are, just as the name suggests, powered manually. Most work with a piston that you pump in order to create suction; however, models such as the Avent Isis and the Medela Harmony use a hand trigger. Many manual pumps do allow the user to vary the suction level. The cycling is determined by your operation. Manual pumps can only be used to pump one breast at a time, but they are convenient to travel with since they are small and compact. However, one drawback of hand pumps is the possibility of repetitive strain injuries to the hand and wrist if used frequently. They can also be awkward to use since both hands are required to hold the pump and the breast, and you are limited in your ability to use hand compressions and massage while pumping.

While there are a few cases in which women have successfully exclusively pumped long term with a manual pump, these success stories are not common. Manual expression is far more time consuming since you are only able to express one breast at a time, and the effort it takes to manually operate the pump will make it more difficult to continue indefinitely. In the vast majority of cases, a manual pump is not an option for exclusively pumping. It may, however, be a useful back-up pump for emergencies or the occasional outing.

Battery Operated and Small Electric Breast Pumps

These pumps are often ones bearing the name of large baby product companies and are most commonly found in drug and department stores. Often, these are the companies that have developed a breast pump in order to offer a complete range of infant products. They most commonly will only allow single-sided pumping and many mothers report that they are uncomfortable to use. While these pumps may be acceptable for infrequent use by a breastfeeding mother, they will not initiate or maintain a milk supply when exclusively pumping.

These pumps are very inexpensive when compared to the better quality single-user pumps or hospital-grade pumps, but do not be seduced by the price—they will not meet your needs and in the end will place your milk supply at risk.

Single-User Double Electric Breast Pumps

There are a number of manufacturers, such as Medela, Ameda, Hygeia, Avent, Spectra, Lansinoh, Limerick, and Bailey Medical, that offer electric breast pumps for single users. This type of pump is intended to be used by only one person and is not intended to be resold or loaned out. Some are closed system pumps and some are open system, and while they are not intended for indefinite and frequent use, as hospital-grade pumps are, most can be an appropriate choice for exclusively pumping mothers.

The most commonly used single-user pumps for exclusively pumping are the Medela Pump in Style Advanced and the Ameda Purely Yours, although in recent years the Hygeia EnJoye has been gaining ground, and the Spectra M1 and Spectra 9 have newly entered the market in North America but have been available in other countries for a longer period. Medela has also added the Freestyle, and the PJ's Bliss by Limerick, the Avent Isis IQ Duo, and the Lansinoh Affinity are other options to consider in this category. Pumps are often rated by the number of hours their motors are expected to perform. This information can help you find the pump that is best suited to the demands of exclusively pumping.

Single-user pumps are compact, lightweight, and portable. Many are built into a carrying case and include cooler compartments, making it very easy to pump on the go. Often this type of pump can also be used with either batteries or a car adapter that can be plugged into the cigarette lighter. Batteries, however, should not be considered as a long-term option. A single pumping session may drain the batteries enough to affect the suction level of the pump. Still, if no other power source is available, the ability to use batteries is a real advantage.

These electric breast pumps can be purchased from numerous stores and from many internet sources. The cost is notably more than the "department store" type of pumps, but their efficiency is far superior. In most cases, this type of pump should be considered the *minimum* needed for exclusively pumping.

Hospital-grade Electric Pumps

The industrial hospital-grade electric pump is the best pump you can use in terms of efficiency, reliability, and durability. These pumps can be cost prohibitive to purchase outright but can be rented at a price that is usually far less than the cost of formula.

And should you decide to purchase one, the cost can actually still be less than formula over the course of a year and these pumps can be resold without concern, making it possible to recoup some of your expenses. Check with your local hospital, health unit, WIC office or health organization to investigate whether they offer subsidized rates for breast pump rentals, and don't forget to check with your insurance company to see if the cost of purchasing a breast pump may be covered. Do be cautious when purchasing a hospital-grade pump though and only buy through a reputable distributor. Rental pumps have been known to find their way onto eBay and other online sales sites and this obviously would leave you, as the consumer, unprotected should you buy from an illegitimate source.

Hospital-grade electric pumps are intended for multiple users and therefore have stronger motors. They also work on a closed system which ensures that milk droplets do not come in contact with the internal workings of the pump, thereby reducing or removing the risk of contamination for all users, and of course allowing a pump to be sold without concern. Each new user should use their own pump kit (flanges and tubing). While this type of pump is not an absolute necessity, it is highly recommended—especially if you are having difficulty building your supply, exclusively pumping from birth, or the mother of a premature baby. You might consider renting a hospital-grade pump for the first two or three months post-partum and then decide if you want to purchase a personal pump or continue with the hospital-grade one.

Hospital-grade electric pumps include such pumps as the Hygeia EnDeare, the Ameda Platinum and Elite, PJ's Comfort by Limerick, the Spectra Dew 350 and S1/S2, and the Medela Lactina and Symphony. The names of breast pumps may differ depending on your location. Some manufacturers will refer to a personal pump as a "hospital-grade" pump, but this is largely marketing.

Unless the pump is intended for multiple users and intended for extended usage (again check the manufacturers' suggested motor life and warranty), it is not truly hospital-grade.

The Bottom Line

Without a doubt, the best pump to use when exclusively pumping is a hospital-grade double electric pump. These pumps not only have the durability to withstand constant use, they are usually the most efficient pumps you can use to remove milk from your breasts. One obvious drawback of these pumps, though, is that they are not readily portable. Yet regardless of your personal situation, the use of a hospital-grade pump will give you the best start possible.

What it comes down to, though, is that the best breast pump is the one that works for you and no one pump will work for every woman. Pumps are different in their design, their comfort, their affordability, and their portability. Consider your needs and make an informed decision. Call around to lactation consultants in your area and see if any offer the opportunity to "test drive" a pump before you purchase. Closed-system pumps will allow for this. If the pump you are using is not comfortable or you notice your supply is not responding favourably, consider trying a different pump. If you purchase a breast pump right from the start, the idea of switching to a different pump if you encounter problems may seem ludicrous. This is another reason why renting a pump at the beginning may be an excellent option. It will allow you to be sure your supply is well established, and also, it will allow you to test the type of pumps available.

Unfortunately, some women will spend money on a pump only to discover it is not living up to its end of the bargain. In these instances, it is important to troubleshoot as much as possible, implement the best pumping practices possible, and consider whether another pump may be the answer. Don't be afraid to switch manufacturers, and don't assume all pumps are the same—find one that works for you! When in doubt, contact the manufacturer. Many provide excellent customer service and will work with you to ensure the pump is operating effectively and meeting your needs.

Breast Pump Checklist

Consider the following questions when deciding on a breast pump that is right for you and your situation:

- Does it need to be portable—will you be travelling with your pump to work or other locations?
- Does the pump fall within the recommended cycling speed (40-60 cycles per minute) and suction levels (up to 200-220 mmHg)?
- Is the pump a closed or open system? Does this matter to you?
- Is the pump a hospital-grade pump or a personal pump? Is this important for your needs?
- What kind of warranty is offered by the manufacturer?
- Are replacement parts (flanges, valves, tubing) easy to find?
- Are a variety of flange sizes available for the pump?
- Are replacement parts expensive or a reasonable cost?
- Does the pump offer a battery backup or a removable manual pump? Do you need this feature?
- Is the pump's manufacturer easy to contact and do they offer online and phone support as well as customer service?

- Has the pump been proven effective by other long-term exclusively pumping mothers?
- Can you use any collection bottle with the pump or do you require specific ones sold by the manufacturer?
- Are you comfortable with the cost?
- Have you checked to see if the cost of the pump can be covered by insurance?
- Have you read through a number of reviews of the pumps you are considering and taken the experience of other users into consideration?
- Is the company WHO Code compliant and responsive to and supportive of breastfeeding mothers? Is this important to you?[14]

Accessories

Flanges

Flanges may also be referred to as horns or breast shields. The flange is the part of the pump that is placed over your breast and nipple and is attached to the tubing. Collection bottles are attached to the flanges. Flanges are usually made out of plastic, although there are some companies that offer softer silicone flanges or silicone inserts as well as extra large glass flanges.

Flanges are available in a number of different sizes allowing a woman to customize them to her particular needs. Some women find they require two different sized flanges. Ensure that the flanges fit you properly. Your nipples should not hit the end of the tube nor should they be squished into the flange. If you find that your nipples are hitting the end or feel that they are squished and you are experiencing discomfort, either while pumping or after your pumping session, consider trying a larger sized flange. Your nipple should move freely within the tunnel of the flange and you should see some movement of the areola — but not too much.

Just as some women will find the standard flanges too small, some women may find the standard flange is too large. Often in this case, a large amount of the areola will be pulled into the flange tube causing excess friction on this part of the breast. If you find sores developing on your areolas, ensure you are using a product such as lanolin, olive oil, or coconut oil to reduce the friction as much as possible. Also, try either smaller flanges, if they are available, or try a silicone insert such as the Ameda Flexishield or the Medela Softfit insert which will reduce the diameter of the flange while providing you with additional comfort. Silicone inserts and flanges are intended to increase the comfort of the mother while pumping as well as to improve let-downs by increasing areola stimulation.

Medela offers the PersonalFit Breastshields. These shields are a two-piece system that allows you to interchange the breast shield to meet your personal needs. The large shield is 27 mm in diameter and the extra large is 30 mm. They also carry an extra large glass breast shield to accommodate even larger nipples. Smaller sizes offered include 25mm, 24mm, and 21mm.

Ameda also offers a wide range of breast shield sizes. Their standard flange size is 25 mm. They also offer a custom flange that is 30.5 mm. With an insert, this custom flange is 28.5 mm in diameter. For smaller nipples, they offer a reducing insert for their standard flange reducing the size to 23 mm and further still to 21 mm if their Flexishield is used.

Hygeia's flanges come in three different sizes. The medium flange is 27mm, large flange is 29mm, and the extra large flange is 31mm.

Not all pump companies offer a variety of flange sizes, so this should be a consideration when deciding on what kind of pump to use. However, another option in flanges is the Pumpin' Pal flange. Pumpin' Pal is an angled flange that can be used with a wide variety of pumps. It is an insert that you use within your pump's original flanges. They are sold in three sizes to accommodate a wide range of women. Anecdotal reports are often very positive towards these flanges.

Hands-free Pumping Bras

Sitting for 120 minutes or more a day, especially when you have a baby to care for, can be challenging. Finding something to do while you are pumping that will allow you to relax, pass the time, and enjoy the time as your own can be complicated by the fact that you need to hold onto the flanges while you pump. Reading, watching television, surfing the internet, or catching up on email are all possible to do when pumping, and it can be nice to have this time for yourself—if your baby will cooperate! For some women though, trying to balance the flanges and bottles with only one hand while attempting to use the other for these pursuits can prove very difficult and frustrating. This is where a hands-free pumping bra can be of use.

There are a few different styles of pumping bras available from a number of manufacturers. Most hands-free pumping bras have slits in the front of the bra into which you slip the flange. Some common hands-free pumping bras include PumpEase, Easy Expression Bustier, Simple Wishes, the Made By Moms pumping band, and Leading Lady. You can readily purchase pumping bras over the internet, and you may even find them at a local department store.

When deciding what kind of pumping bra you want to purchase, be sure to carefully consider how well it will stand up to frequent use. Consider the method the bra uses to hold the pump flanges. You do not want the bra to stretch and no longer hold the flanges tightly to your breast. You will also want it to be convenient, easy, and quick to use.

Another option is to make a pumping bra. Some women simply take an old, snug-fitting bra and cut slits into it for the flanges to fit into. You may find the holes you cut do stretch over time though, and this might be reason enough to purchase a bra designed especially for pumping. If you have a sewing machine, simply zigzag stitching around the opening can give it some added stability. If you have a serger, even better.

While not a necessity for exclusively pumping, a hands-free pumping bra can allow you to pass the time without staring at your collection bottles. It may even allow you to enjoy your time pumping and use it as much deserved personal time.

Pump, Kit, and Collection System Maintenance

Collecting and storing breast milk is quite simple and by following some basic guidelines you will soon get into the groove and create a routine that works for you. As with any food handling, it is important to keep items used to collect and store your milk clean. This is most important for premature, ill, or very young babies. As we all know, eventually babies get bigger, start exploring their world, and touching and tasting everything in sight—and as mothers we tend to also relax our cleaning and sterilizing routines. This holds true when exclusively pumping, and you'll likely find you are washing and sterilizing more often in the early weeks.

Follow these guidelines in addition to the instructions provided with your pump:

- Wash your hands before handling your pump kit or using your pump.
- Wipe down your pump before and after each use.
- Cover your pump, or keep it in its case, when not using it to protect it from dust and debris.

- Inspect the pump regularly for signs of wear or damage.
- Inspect the tubing regularly for signs of wear, punctures, condensation, or mold. Replace the tubing if necessary. Tubing may get condensation in it. If this happens, try running your pump with the tubing attached for a couple minutes to dry it out. If you notice mold in the tubing, replace it. With the open system pumps, you may discover milk has backed up into the tubing. While this is not common, it can happen. While you can rinse the tubing and hang it to dry, it is better to simply replace the tubing to ensure you are using parts that are as clean as possible, especially given the fact that the cost of additional tubing is minimal.
- The valves and membranes on the pump kit deserve special attention. All valves and membranes will wear and can tear. It is good preventative maintenance to replace them regularly—at least every two or three months. They are inexpensive and can make an enormous difference in the effectiveness of your pump. Keep extra valves or membranes on hand in case the ones you are using get damaged.
- Dismantle your pump on a regular schedule and clean it thoroughly. Depending on the type of pump you are using, you will be able to dismantle it to varying degrees. Refer to the owner's manual or ask the rental station. If you are using the Pump in Style, be sure to remove the face plate regularly and clean behind it. Cleaning is best done with a clean, damp cloth. Avoid using

harsh chemicals or detergents, especially on any part that comes in contact with milk.

- Dismantle and clean your pump kit every time you pump (although some alternatives to this are coming up). Since the pump kit is the part of the pump with which the breast milk comes in direct contact, it should perhaps be given the most attention. It is best to take it apart: remove all removable parts and wash each one in hot, soapy water. Rinse each part well and allow to air dry. Once dry, either cover with a clean cloth or place in a clean container or plastic storage bag.

- One alternative to cleaning pump kits after each use is to simply place the kit in a plastic storage bag and store it in the refrigerator until the next pumping session. Since expressed breast milk can safely be kept at room temperature for several hours and will keep in the fridge for a number of days, keeping the flanges in the fridge follows the same guidelines. This can certainly reduce the amount of time required for cleaning and make pumping, especially in the early months, more manageable. This time-saving strategy should only be used if your baby is healthy and full-term, and you will want to ensure you disassemble the pump kit and clean it thoroughly once a day (perhaps a good job for daddy?).

- Another option is to buy more than one pump kit. This will reduce the frequency of washing.

- For ill or premature babies, pump kits should be sterilized according to your hospital's recommendations. As a general guideline, pumps should be sterilized after each use if you are pumping at the hospital. When at home, it is best to sterilize at least once daily.

- If your own immunity has been compromised by a yeast infection, you should sterilize your equipment after each use.

Sterilization of your pump kit should be done before its first use. You can sterilize in an open pot of boiling water or use a steam sterilizer. A steam sterilizer can be a very quick and time-conserving method to sterilize kits.

The Human Milk Banking Association of North America (HMBANA) does not consider it necessary to sterilize pumps regularly, provided you are washing the pump kit thoroughly and on a regular basis.[15] However, other sources suggest that dishwasher sterilization should at least be used to ensure bacterial contamination is kept to a minimum.[16] To make cleaning easy and to benefit from added sterilization, you may be able to run your pump kit through the dishwasher. Check with the pump company to see if this is possible. Although sterilization may not be necessary on a frequent basis for full-term healthy infants once they have reached a few months of age, I still think it is good practice to sterilize the pump kit every few days.

Since the breast pump you use is important to initiate and maintain your supply, take good care of it. Regular cleaning and maintenance will ensure your milk is able to be stored in a safe manner, for a longer period, and will also ensure that the breast pump works as efficiently as possible for as long as possible.

Chapter 9

Feeding Baby

So you've expressed your milk and your baby is ready to eat. Here's where you reap the rewards of all your hard work and dedication! Exclusively pumping brings with it a unique set of requirements. Not only do you need to deal with bottles and nipples and cleaning—as you would if you were formula feeding—but you also need to understand breast milk storage. There are similarities between feeding formula and feeding expressed breast milk as far as the devices used, but breast milk is a special food and learning a bit about how to store and feed it will ensure your baby receives all the good stuff you are working so hard for. If you do your own research you will find that recommendations for the use and storage of expressed breast milk do vary; however, there are basic guidelines and ranges of storage times that are most commonly viewed as appropriate and in this chapter we'll discuss those. Sometimes feeding expressed breast milk becomes unnecessarily complex and mothers who have worked so hard for that milk worry that they'll do something wrong or somehow "ruin" the milk they have expressed. Set your fears aside. Use your best judgment, work within the guidelines, and rest assured that your milk is exactly what your baby needs.

Collection Bottles

Collection bottles are the bottles you will attach to the breast pump and express milk into. Just about any plastic or glass baby bottle will fit onto the major brands of breast pumps. The only exception is wide mouth bottles. However, you can purchase conversion kits which will allow you to use wide mouth bottles with many different pump brands.

Pumping directly into feeding bottles can be especially useful if you are going to feed your baby shortly after you pump since you can simply attach a nipple and feed without needing to transfer into another bottle or warm the milk. Your baby will also get as much of the "good stuff" as possible when feeding freshly expressed milk. However, if you are going to store the breast milk in the refrigerator, it is best to use collection bottles with tight fitting lids such as the ones that come with most breast pumps. You can also purchase these separately, and you can never have too many collection bottles.

Ensure that collection bottles are carefully cleaned. While bottles should be sterilized for a pre-term or ill infant, you may simply wash them in hot soapy water for full-term, healthy infants.

There are numerous places to purchase bottles to use for milk collection. Any department or drug store will sell common brands of baby bottles. Bottles made specifically for expressed milk can be purchased from any number of online stores selling breast pumps and accessories, and you can usually find them in local department stores or baby stores. Also, check with your local health unit and hospital to see if they sell pumps and accessories or if they can refer you to a local business where you can purchase these supplies.

Another consideration when deciding on collection bottles is the size of the bottle. Most bottles made for expressed breast milk collection are four-ounce bottles. Some baby bottles are four or five ounces, but many are eight or nine ounces in size. When your supply increases you may find you do sometimes need to switch bottles part way through a pumping session if you are using four-ounce collection bottles and you may therefore find that larger bottles are more convenient. In the beginning, however, four-ounce bottles should be more than adequate. Women with shorter torsos may find the larger bottles more cumbersome and difficult to handle due to their length.

Depending on your long-term storage requirements, use what works for you. There is no need to spend significant amounts of money on collection bottles, especially if you are not planning on using them to freeze or store long term in your refrigerator.

Containers for Fridge and Freezer Storage

So once you've expressed the milk, what do you do with it? There are a number of different options and what is best for your situation will depend on a number of factors: amount of milk being stored, cost, where you are storing the milk, and how long you plan to pump. In general, choose the best, most protective containers you can afford, but don't over-think it. Each type of storage system has its pros and cons.

There is some disagreement on whether glass or plastic bottles are better for milk storage. The "best" depends on how you are storing the breast milk. Clear, hard plastic bottles made of polycarbonate that have tight fitting lids are often considered the best choice for short-term storage in the refrigerator since live cells such as leukocytes (white cells which fight infection) have been shown to stick to glass; however, some later research suggests the length of storage is more significant than the type of container.[1,2] The Academy of Breastfeeding Medicine states that glass and polypropylene containers "appear similar in their effects on adherence of lipid-soluble nutrients to the container's surface, the concentration of immunoglobulin A, and the numbers of viable white blood cells in the stored milk."[3] If you are storing milk in the refrigerator for more than a day, glass or plastic may not matter. Cell counts in glass containers increase after a 24-hour period and it would seem that this is a result of the cells releasing from the glass. Freezing destroys live cells, so the fact that leukocytes stick to glass is not a concern when freezing breast milk in glass containers.

Glass might be considered as the best choice for freezer storage since it is non-porous and protects IgA antibodies and other proteins. However, glass bottles for freezing can be difficult to find. Plastic bottles are also an acceptable alternative and rigid polypropylene bottles have been shown to maintain the stability of cells.[4] If you decide to freeze in glass bottles, you can use baby food jars or small mason jars. Both of these options can be cost effective if you have a supply on hand or know of someone who does. Be sure to sterilize the jars and lids before using them. Another benefit of glass jars is that they can easily be sterilized and reused. Remember that the milk will expand when frozen, so always leave a bit of empty space at the top of the jar, and always check to ensure the integrity of the glass before you use the milk. Occasionally, glass will crack in the freezer.

When freezing expressed breast milk, it is best to freeze in small amounts in order to reduce waste if the entire portion is not eaten or needed once it is thawed. However, if you have large amounts of breast milk to freeze, this may not always be an option due to the expense of storage containers.

Another popular option for storage is plastic storage bags specifically designed for expressed breast milk. Polyethylene bags have been shown to reduce the amount of IgA antibodies by as much as 60%, but ease of storage may win out.[5, 6] Medela,

Ameda, Gerber, Bailey Medical, Lansinoh, Hygeia, Avent, Honeysuckle, and Simplisse all make bags for breast milk storage. There are a number of benefits of breast milk storage bags compared to other freezer bags:

- pre-sterilized
- made of thicker plastic to protect from freezer burn and odours in freezer
- some are multi-ply
- some are also lined with nylon to prevent fat from sticking to the sides of the bag
- many have a zipper-type seal which helps to prevent leakage
- some fit onto pump kits.

Not all breast milk storage bags are created equal, so do your own research to determine which one is best for you. Bags also are notorious for leaking when thawed. Not all bags leak, but they will definitely leak more than bottles will. When thawing bags of milk, place the bag into a clean bowl or plastic container in case the bag does have a tear. This will prevent you from losing the milk—and prevent a mess in your kitchen. Storage bags have a couple benefits over using glass or plastic bottles:

- quicker to thaw
- freezing flat can make better use of valuable freezer space.

Another option for freezing expressed breast milk is to use other types of plastic bags: freezer bags or bottle liners. Freezer bags are better since they have a sealed closure that will better prevent leaks. Bottle liners should be doubled to provide a stronger barrier, but know that since this type of bag must be closed using twist ties it is more likely to lead to leakage or spillage of milk than some other types of storage systems. With either type of bag, store several smaller bags inside a larger freezer bag to help prevent leaks and provide an extra barrier to protect the milk in the freezer.

One final method you might consider is exceptionally simple. Freeze breast milk in ice cube trays and once it is frozen, pop out the cubes and store in plastic freezer bags. This allows you to take out of the freezer as much, or as little, milk as you need. The small cubes make it easier to thaw, and they are easily portable. There are a number of tray systems on the market, but you can simply use regular ice cube trays as well.

The type of storage containers you do want to avoid are those made with bisphenol A (BPA). This chemical has been identified as an endocrine disruptor. Some countries, such as Canada, have a ban on bisphenol A being used in any baby product, but it is best to check and ensure the plastic you are using is indeed free of it.

Feeding Bottles

If you will not be breastfeeding at all, then use any bottle and nipple your baby likes. You may prefer to use a silicone nipple since they last longer and are easier to clean. You may also consider using an orthodontic type nipple.

If you are still working to establish breastfeeding, or if you continue to breastfeed for comfort, then you may choose to use a wide-mouth bottle and nipple. This type of nipple will encourage your baby to use a wider latch. Using a slow flow nipple will also continue to make your baby work for her milk and not get her used to the fast, easy flow of other nipples.

Using a slow flow nipple is best regardless of whether you are breastfeeding or not, as many babies have difficulty with the quick flow of milk from the faster flow nipples. Since milk is always flowing from a bottle nipple, babies have no ability to slow down or stop the flow if they need a break and a slow flow nipple will allow them a more comfortable pace when feeding. As your baby gets older you may want to switch to a faster flow nipple.

If your baby suffers from severe colic or reflux, you may want to use a bottle that can reduce these symptoms. Look for bottles that limit the amount of air entering the milk. From personal experience with a baby who suffered from reflux, I can attest to the fact that this type of bottle can have a positive impact.

Paced bottle feeding should, ideally, be practiced by anyone bottle feeding any baby and is discussed later in the chapter.

Pumping and Storing Expressed Breast Milk

For ease of use and to keep as much bioactivity in the milk as possible, freshly expressed breast milk is best to use whenever possible. This may not always be practical, but it can make life much easier to simply pump and feed without having to warm the milk or worry about using the "older" milk first.

If necessary, you can also pump directly into previously expressed milk that has been stored at room temperature as long as it is less than eight hours old. You should then use this milk for your baby's next feeding. It is best to cool down freshly expressed milk before adding it to refrigerated milk, and you can add chilled milk to previously frozen milk provided the amount you are adding is less than the amount frozen.[7] So many options!

It's a good idea to keep track of the date and time you express your milk. While not as important to label milk in the fridge since usually you'll only have a few bottles in the fridge at a time and it is easier to organize it from oldest to newest, it *is* important to label milk going into the freezer. Doing this will help you keep track of the milk you have and ensure you use your oldest milk first (if not feeding fresh milk) and rotate your frozen stash as needed. Depending on the containers you use for milk storage, you can label with marker, wax pencil, sticky labels, or even tape. Just be sure whatever method you choose will stay affixed during storage and doesn't leach into the milk through the container.

Effects of Storage

It is important to start this section off by emphasizing that all breast milk has important properties and even though storage will reduce its effects to some extent, you should be confident that your milk is always the right choice for your baby. Many moms want to know just how storage affects their milk though, so in this section we'll look at some of the research.

The cell function of expressed milk has been shown to decrease the longer it is stored. Temperature also has an impact on stored milk. The concentration of normal flora in breast milk actually decreases over time after it has been expressed due to the activity of the bacterial inhibiting factors of the milk, and these elements remain active during both refrigeration and freezing. Pasteurization of milk destroys these properties.[8]

When specifically considering storage at room temperature, or outside of a fridge or freezer, digestive enzymes, lipase, and amylase levels remain stable over a 24-hour period at environmental temperatures ranging from 15°C to 38°C. Bacterial growth remains low at lower temperatures, but begins to increase when temperatures also increase and is quite high once temperatures are in the range of 38 °C, when the milk is stored for 4 to 8 hours. This is important to know if you live in a warm area without air conditioning in the summer months. When temperatures rise above 25°C, it is best to put any unused milk into the fridge.[9]

Most refrigerators maintain a temperature of 0-4°C. This temperature range will significantly slow bacterial growth and the cellular activity of breast milk is also greatly reduced at this temperature. Refrigeration that exceeds 48 hours has been shown to result in a 50% decrease of viable and functional cells, so your best option is to use fresh or to freeze what you don't need as soon as possible.[10] Creamatocrit levels (a method of determining fat and caloric content of milk) decrease if milk is stored at room temperature, but remain stable at refrigerator temperatures. The breakdown of fat decreases in milk stored at 25°C and 4°C and increases at higher temperatures.[11]

Freezing doesn't introduce any new bacterial changes to the milk, and bacterial fighting activity has been shown to remain in milk frozen for as long as three weeks.[12] Freezing doesn't introduce any new changes in milk's composition with the exception of the breakdown of fat, demulsification, and the breakdown of proteins when the milk is thawed. After freezing, fat may also stick to the sides of the container and be difficult to remove.[13] Freezing has only a minimal effect on antibodies, but greatly affects cellular stability. No live cells remain in milk after it has been frozen.[14]

General Guidelines for Storing Breast Milk

Once you've been pumping for awhile, you will become an expert in the use and storage of expressed breast milk. In the meantime, here are some basic guidelines to consider:

- Store in small amounts (two to four ounces) when possible. This is most important when your baby is young and taking relatively small amounts of milk per feed.
- Milk expands when frozen, so ensure you leave sufficient room in the container to allow for expansion—about an inch should be enough. This is especially important if using glass containers.

- Write the date and amount of expressed breast milk on each storage container.
- There is some concern with using permanent marker on plastic bags due to the possibility of the marker leaching into the milk. Some manufacturers avoid this risk by placing the labeling area outside of the bag's storage chamber. To avoid this problem with other bags, use self-adhesive labels.
- Freeze bags of milk flat. Once frozen, you may stack them or, better yet, place a number of bags into a larger freezer bag for storage. One woman who contacted me had an ingenious method of storing frozen bags of breast milk. She cut a small opening in the side of a gift bag, down near the bottom of the bag, and placed the frozen bags of milk horizontally in the bag. The opening in the bottom of the bag allows you to slip one bag out at a time while keeping the rest of the bags neat and orderly. Simple and effective!
- Reorganize your expressed breast milk in the refrigerator and freezer often, keeping the newest milk at the bottom or back of the freezer and bringing the oldest milk to the top or the front. Be sure to always use the oldest milk first.
- Check your freezer regularly to ensure it is operating properly. Be sure everyone in your family understands how important it is to keep the freezer door closed.
- Keep milk stored in the fridge towards the back of the compartment and away from the door to prevent temperature variation. If storing milk in

a refrigerator freezer, keep it towards the back and keep the freezer closed as much as possible.

- If you are storing expressed breast milk in a fridge at work or in someone else's home, it is best to label it as expressed breast milk. Both to prevent any unnecessary accidents, contamination, or inadvertent use. You don't want a co-worker finding out the hard way!

Storage Times

If you look at three different sources of information providing safe storage times for expressed breast milk, you'll likely come away with three different sets of guidelines. What is important to realize is that they are just that: guidelines. Use the guidelines and your judgment, taking into consideration your baby's needs, health, and the environmental temperature. We do know that the temperature at which expressed milk is stored does have an effect on its safety. Yet, as the Academy of Breastfeeding Medicine points out in its clinical protocol, there is as of yet no definition of "unsafe milk" that has been agreed upon.[15] In general terms, it is best to always use expressed breast milk as soon as possible, refrigerate it as soon as possible, and freeze it if it will not be used within twenty-four to forty-eight hours.

Here is a review of the most common breast milk storage guidelines:

- Room temperature (16-29°C; 60-85°F): up to 8 hours. 3-4 hours is considered optimal and 6-8 hours should be used only when very clean conditions exist. At this temperature, there is a minimal loss of nutrients and protective properties.

- Refrigerator (4°C; 39°F): up to 8 days. Less than 3 days is considered optimal and longer than that should be used only when very clean conditions exist. At this temperature and for this length of storage time, most elements remain intact and there is limited bacteria in the milk.
- Freezer (-20°C; 0°F): up to 12 months, with 6 months considered optimal. Frozen milk will have reduced cell count and activity, as well as changes to fat globules and protein. If milk is stored in a refrigerator freezer it should be used within 3 to 4 months.[16]

Using Fresh Milk

- If you are feeding expressed breast milk, leave out only enough milk for your baby's next feeding and refrigerate or freeze the rest.
- Be aware of environmental conditions. When it is particularly hot, room temperature storage times will be reduced. Always best to err on the side of caution.
- Always smell and perhaps even taste the milk before feeding to be sure it has not soured, especially if it has been sitting out for awhile. Usually smelling it will be enough to determine if it is okay, but if it is in question, you might consider tasting it as well.
- Freshly pumped milk can make going out on a trip to the grocery store, the park, or out to lunch much easier since you will not need to worry about cooling the milk after expressing as long as you will be using it within a couple hours. You

will also not need to warm the milk since it will be kept at room temperature and most babies will happily accept milk at room temperature.

Using Refrigerated Milk

- Always use the oldest refrigerated expressed breast milk first.
- There is a limited amount of research that shows breast milk can be refrigerated for up to eight days at 0-4°C (32-39°F). If you are pumping more than your baby requires, it is good practice to freeze any excess breast milk on a daily basis.
- Smell and taste the milk before feeding to ensure it has not soured.
- You can warm the milk, although some people choose not to and some babies don't seem to mind cold milk. It can, however, be gentler on little tummies to warm the milk.
- Gently swirl the milk to mix in any separated fat. Shaking can break down the proteins in breast milk. In this case you want it "stirred not shaken". Sorry, Mr. Bond.

Using Frozen Milk

- Always use the oldest milk first to extend the life of your freezer stash.
- The best way to thaw breast milk is to refrigerate it. Depending on your storage container, this can take anywhere from twelve to twenty-four hours. If using milk storage bags, place them in a bowl or in a larger bag in case the storage bag leaks.

- You can place the frozen milk in a container of warm water or run under cool water until thawed.
- If you use heat to thaw milk, you should use it right away.
- Once thawed, provided this is done without the use of heat, breast milk can be kept in the refrigerator for up to twenty-four hours. After being frozen and thawed, breast milk's ability to inhibit bacterial growth is greatly compromised, so treat it carefully and do not leave it out at room temperature for more than a few hours.[17] Thawed breast milk tends to be much more fragile and you may find it deteriorates quickly. It may not last twenty-four hours after thawing.
- While it may be best not to refreeze thawed milk, one study does suggest milk that has been thawed in the refrigerator for up to eight hours may be safely refrozen.[18] Since this is only one study, the results should be considered cautiously.
- Once milk has been warmed and fed to your baby, it should be used up within one to two hours or discarded.[19]

Warming Expressed Breast Milk

To warm cold breast milk, you can place it in a container of warm water until it reaches room temperature or slightly warmer. You can also use a bottle warmer. Do not use boiling water.

Never heat breast milk on the stove or in a microwave. Not only can this cause hot spots in the milk that can scald the baby, but it can also destroy vital properties in the milk.[20] Always test the temperature of the milk after gently mixing it and before feeding it to your baby.

Feeding Expressed Breast Milk

One of the most common questions asked by new moms who are feeding expressed breast milk is "How much should my baby be eating?" This question is both easy and difficult to answer. It's easy because you simply want to feed your baby as much as he wants. But it's difficult in the sense that when bottle feeding, a baby doesn't have as much control over intake as he would if breastfeeding. Research has shown that there are behavioural differences between bottle-fed and breastfed babies.[21] A breastfed baby can stop actively sucking and the milk flow will slow or stop. A bottle nipple doesn't work this way though. Even slow flow bottle nipples will continually drip or stream milk when the bottle is inclined. This is concern number one.

The second problem comes with babies' intrinsic need to suck. It's what babies are born to do and they need to fulfill this instinct. Some babies have a much greater need to suck than others, and if their only opportunity to meet this need comes when they are being bottle fed, then this will sometimes result in overfeeding.

As will be discussed in more detail in the chapter "Pumping and the NICU", there are some helpful guidelines to be aware of when it comes to monitoring your baby's intake. Counting wet and dirty diapers is a good way to monitor your baby's intake. If it goes in, it has to come out, right? You should see one wet and dirty diaper per day of life for the first three days after your baby is born (so a one-day old will have one wet and one dirty diaper, a two day old will have two wet and two dirty diapers, etc.). After day three your baby should have three or four stooled diapers each day, with the colour transitioning from black meconium to softer, yellow stools. Stooling patterns will sometimes change after a few weeks for babies receiving breast milk and several days may pass between stooling. As long as your baby isn't in discomfort or straining to pass the bowel movement, there is no concern. After a couple days of life your baby should continue to have about five to six wet diapers a day.

The other way to tell that your baby is getting enough is to monitor her weight. Babies should regain their birth weight by ten days of age and should gain about 5-7 ounces per week (170 grams/week). Weight gain will usually slow down around three months of age to 4-5 ounces per week (113-142 grams/week), and again around six months of age to about 2-4 ounces per week (57-113 grams/week).

Keep track of your baby's growth using World Health Organization growth charts for breastfed babies. Weight patterns vary significantly between breastfed and formula-fed infants. You can download these growth charts for your own use from the WHO website.[22]

Here are some other points to consider when feeding expressed breast milk:

- Use the feeding bottle of your choice. Vented bottles might be helpful for babies with reflux or digestive troubles, but generally, unless you're working to transition to breastfeeding, the bottle choice is up to you.
- Feed on cue instead of on a schedule. Look for cues such as restlessness, mouthing, licking lips, lip smacking, and rooting. Remember that crying is a very late hunger cue and it's better to catch the earlier cues.
- Do not encourage your baby to finish every bottle if he seems like he has had enough. Although controversial at the moment, many believe

breastfeeding may reduce the incidence of obesity. This may be a benefit of breast milk itself;
however, it may also be due to the baby's ability
to self-regulate his intake when at the breast. For
this reason, allow your baby to determine how
much milk he needs.[23, 24]

- As just mentioned, some babies will overeat simply to satisfy their need to suck. If your baby is
  noticeably uncomfortable after eating large
  amounts, or spitting up large amounts of milk,
  offer a pacifier and see if this will satisfy him.
- Average intake will be around 750 milliliters (25
  ounces) per day with boys being slightly higher
  in their intake.[25]
- Intake will slowly decline after the introduction
  of solids as solid meals start to replace the required calories.

Paced Bottle Feeding

Paced bottle feeding, sometimes referred to as bottle nursing, is a
means of bottle feeding that more closely follows normal
breastfeeding behaviours. Breastfeeding provides a great deal of
interaction between a mom and baby and also provides a baby
with a great deal of control over how often to nurse and how
much milk she drinks; it is hypothesized that the lack of this
control may be responsible—at least in part—for the increased
risk of obesity in bottle fed children. But bottle feeding doesn't
mean you can't include the same type of interactions as are
normally seen with breastfeeding, just as breastfeeding doesn't
ensure these interactions will take place. What is important is
your ability and desire to respond to your baby and be aware of
the cues and signals she uses to communicate her needs. Some of
the key aspects of paced bottle feeding include the following:

- Allow the baby to draw the bottle nipple into his or her mouth instead of forcing or placing the nipple into the mouth.
- Feed according to normal, early-feeding cues as opposed to feeding on a schedule.
- Hold the bottle in a horizontal position. Tilt it vertically only enough to keep milk in the nipple.
- Hold your baby in an upright position. Do not recline the baby during feeding.
- Switch sides during the feeding session. If you start by holding your baby in your left arm, end the feeding holding your baby in your right arm.
- Pace the feeding so that it lasts 10-20 minutes. Do not allow your baby to guzzle the bottle.
- Take frequent breaks during the feeding session. Just as a nursing baby has periods of active nursing and rest, a bottle-fed baby will benefit from frequent breaks when feeding. Rest the bottle nipple on the baby's chin or cheek during the break and then allow the baby to draw the nipple back into his or her mouth when ready to resume feeding.
- Allow the baby to indicate fullness. Do not encourage a baby to finish a bottle.[26]

The Look and Smell of Expressed Breast Milk

Fresh

Breast milk may have a slightly bluish colouration. The colour of breast milk can change depending on the mother's diet or medication she may take. Breast milk is rather thin, but this does not have a direct relationship to the fat content of the milk. It usually has no noticeable smell and has a slightly sweet taste.

Refrigerated

Breast milk that has been stored in the refrigerator has the same colour and taste as fresh milk. It will separate with a layer of fatty cream forming at the top. The fat may also form into clumps. The fat can be gently mixed into the milk before being fed to the baby. Expressed breast milk can take on the smells of other foods in the fridge. Keep an open box of baking soda in the fridge to limit this. Also, use quality storage containers and avoid keeping strong smelling foods such as onions in the fridge.

Frozen

After thawing, breast milk will be the same colour as fresh or refrigerated breast milk. Some slight variation is possible. The smell and taste of frozen milk can be altered by freezing. If your milk smells rancid, it is best not to use it. If you find you are having difficulties with long-term storage of your milk, you might consider adding probiotics to your diet, changing your drinking water, taking antioxidants (such as vitamin A and E), and investigating the type of fats you are eating. Sometimes changes such as these can alter your breast milk in such a way that the storage problem is resolved. Women sometimes report a soapy or metallic smell to thawed breast milk. The taste may also reflect the smell. It is thought that this is a result of lipase activity in the milk. Generally, if your baby accepts the milk, it is fine to use. If your baby refuses it, however, you may need to make some changes. The next section discusses high lipase and steps to counteract it if necessary.

Lipase—Too much of a good thing

Lipase is a component of milk that does great things. Lipase aids in breaking down the fat in breast milk. For women with very high lipase levels, expressed breast milk may, after sitting for a while or after a longer period of storage in the freezer, begin to smell soapy. The smell is simply a result of lipase doing its job. In effect, the milk is being digested and fats are being broken down. As long as the milk is not sour, it is okay to feed. Many babies will not notice the smell and will accept the milk without concern. If your baby does not accept the milk, you may need to take some extra steps to preserve your breast milk.

To limit the effects of lipase, you can scald your breast milk briefly on the stove prior to storing it. Heat it on a low heat just until small bubbles break the surface, but do not boil the milk. Heating milk to above 40°C will result in the loss of enzyme activity and should be avoided.[27] Allow the milk to cool in the pot and then you can use it right away, store it in the fridge, or freeze it following the usual guidelines. The following are some things you might consider trying if you're having difficulties with high lipase levels:

- Try freezing breast milk in a different type of container.
- Avoid the use of a self-defrosting freezer if possible since the thaw/freeze of the defrost cycle may affect the breast milk. If this is not possible, try to not store the breast milk next to the walls of the freezer.[28]
- Change your thawing method.
- Reduce the length of time you are storing the milk after thawing it. Thawed breast milk is quite fragile and tends to deteriorate more quickly.
- Scald your milk before freezing it.
- Cool your milk before freezing it, or freeze it directly after being pumped.
- Try increasing your antioxidant levels through either diet or supplementation. This might make the fat less susceptible to lipase activity.[29]

Supplementing With Formula

Some women will never require any type of intervention or alternative strategies for increasing or maintaining their milk supply. They pump, and they produce ample amounts of milk for their baby's daily needs with enough left over to build up a significant freezer stash. However, some women will not find a sufficient supply so easy to come by. It's not always possible to know where you will fall in the supply "lottery", but if supply is a concern, then it's okay to supplement with formula. That's what formula is there for and it should be seen as a lifesaving alternative when enough breast milk is not available.

While most women who exclusively pump want to provide 100% breast milk for their babies, this is not always possible. There are many factors that come into play when initiating milk supply: some within your control and some not. In some cases, supplementation with commercially prepared formula will be necessary.

When supplementing with formula, it is best to feed bottles of breast milk and bottles of formula separately. There are a number of reasons for this:

- The anti-infective properties of breast milk may be reduced by combining it with formula.[30]
- Iron from other sources—solids as well as formula—can affect a baby's ability to absorb iron from breast milk. Iron in breast milk is present in lower quantities than infant formula, but it is much more bioavailable, meaning that your baby can use it to a greater extent. Iron in breast milk bonds to lactoferrin, a protein in breast milk, and this is important for two reasons. The first is that lactoferrin can easily pass through a baby's gut so the iron gets into the baby's bloodstream. The

second is that by binding to lactoferrin, the iron is prevented from being used by pathogens in a baby's gut and instead is used for the baby's growth. It is possible that an overload of iron from other food sources saturates the lactoferrin in breast milk and prevents it from serving its many other roles including antiviral, antimicrobial, anti-inflammatory, and supporting the wider immune system.[31, 32]

- The beneficial effects of lysozyme, an antimicrobial factor of breast milk, have been shown to be reduced when cow's milk-based formula or soy-based formula is added to breast milk.[33]

- Once you mix breast milk and formula, you must then treat it as you would formula, which means if it is not finished within two hours, it must be discarded. For women who are struggling to produce every drop, it can be heartbreaking to throw out any amount of breast milk. In this case, feed breast milk and formula separately.

But let's be realistic: sometimes you need to mix the two, and you should know that there is *no* danger in doing so. It is perfectly safe and sometimes may be necessary or preferred. Mixing formula and breast milk is also a helpful method of switching a baby onto formula when weaning.

When using formula, it is important to follow safe handling guidelines. Formula and expressed breast milk are not equivalent when it comes to handling. The World Health Organization has created a report on safe infant formula practices.[34] This is a great place to start, but it's important to realize that safe handling varies depending on where you live, the quality of your water, and the age and health of your baby.

If your baby was born prematurely, born with a low birth weight, or is immuno-compromised for any reason, it is important to be extra vigilant. It is recommended that a sterile, ready-mixed, liquid infant formula be used for such infants. If you can't use the sterile, liquid formula, then you can use powdered formula using the following process. After boiling and then cooling the water to about 70 degrees C (158 degrees F), pour the water into sterilized bottles and mix with the appropriate amount of formula powder. Always be careful to use correct amounts, as formula that is too dilute or too concentrated can affect the health of a baby. The use of hot water to prepare formula is recommended by the WHO as a way to ensure no *Enterobacter sakazakii* is present. *Enterobacter sakazakii* causes bloodstream and central nervous system infections, and although rare, it has been found in infant formula in the past. Once the formula has cooled to an appropriate temperature for your baby, you can feed it right away. Any formula not used immediately should be kept in the fridge and used within 24 hours, or else discarded. Once you have started feeding from a bottle of formula it must be used within two hours or thrown away.

For full-term, healthy infants, follow the above guidelines for preparing infant formula if you wish to prepare it ahead of time and keep it in the fridge until you need it. If you want to prepare one bottle at a time for immediate use, you can use previously boiled and cooled water that has been keep in a sterile container.

To warm infant formula you can place the bottle in a warm cup of water or in a bottle warmer. It is never a good idea to warm bottles in a microwave as it can cause hot spots that may scald your baby's mouth.

As your baby gets older, you'll likely begin to relax the process of formula preparation, but always keep your water source in mind. For example, if you live in a rural area and use water from a well, it may be best to continue sterilizing the water for a longer period of time,[35] and it's always a good idea to test your well water regularly to ensure its safety for your entire family.

There is absolutely no reason to be discouraged about supplementing with formula. Many mothers supplement at one time or another—both pumping mothers and breastfeeding mothers. Keep working on increasing your supply, but recognize that your baby is still benefiting from your dedication to pump and that every drop of breast milk your baby receives provides great benefit.

Other Common Situations

Freezer Failure/Power Outages

Unfortunately, power outages and freezer failures are a possibility. It is best to be prepared and have a plan in place to either guard against these situations or know how to deal with them if they do arise.

Be sure to regularly check your freezer to ensure it is operating properly. If you find that it has failed, check all of the milk immediately. Any that is still frozen should be put into a cooler with ice or freezer packs and transferred to a working freezer as soon as possible. You can also use as much as possible within the next twenty-four to thirty-six hours depending on how long ago your freezer failed. As long as there are still ice crystals in the milk it is okay to put it back into a working freezer and refreeze.

If you have a power outage, cover your freezer with blankets to add insulation and keep in the cold. Do not open the freezer unless absolutely necessary. The contents of the freezer should stay frozen for at least forty-eight hours if it is full (always keep your freezer as full as possible since it will work more efficiently this way). Once power has been restored, check the frozen milk carefully. The milk stored on the outside of the freezer is most vulnerable.

Traveling Long Distances with Frozen Milk

If you are moving or travelling and need to transport frozen breast milk, the best way to do this is to pack it in a cooler with dry ice and newspaper. Check your local yellow pages or online to find a supplier of dry ice.

On the Go with Expressed Breast Milk

Getting out of the house can sometimes seem like quite the challenge when you are pumping, but going out with expressed breast milk can actually be quite easy. If you pump just before you leave, you can take that fresh milk with you. It will be fine for a few hours depending on the temperature. Check the storage guidelines provided previously in this chapter.

If the day is very hot, or the milk has been previously cooled, you can use a portable cooler bag with ice packs to keep the milk chilled. To warm the milk you have several options:

- Run it under hot tap water.
- Ask for a cup of warm water from a restaurant.
- Bring a thermos of hot water with you to warm the bottle.
- Warm the bottle between your hands or thighs to take the chill off of it.
- Take the bottle of milk out of the cooler 10-15 minutes before feeding to allow it to warm up slightly.
- Feed the milk cold. Some babies will not mind the occasional cold bottle.

As you get more comfortable with pumping and feeding, you'll begin to develop your own timesaving techniques and find what works best for you and your family. There is no one right way to do this. Take the ideas that work, connect with other exclusively pumping moms to see what's working for them, and experiment to see what fits your lifestyle the best.

Chapter 10

Pumping and the NICU

No one ever expects to have a baby in the neonatal intensive care unit (NICU). When suddenly faced with this reality you are often completely overwhelmed and may even be in a state of shock. Whatever expectations you had for your pregnancy and delivery end with a hard landing in the NICU—a world of tubes, machines, monitors, isolettes, gowns and masks, and medical staff who often forget that you are a new mother wondering how you ended up here. And then comes another reality: breastfeeding is going to take a different shape as well. You may have planned on breastfeeding your new baby, or perhaps you've been encouraged to pump even though breastfeeding wasn't something you ever thought you'd do. Now with your little one in the hospital and perhaps fighting his own health battles, you find a new path ahead of you and your role immeasurably changed from the one you expected.

Many babies are in the NICU because they were born prematurely, although stays in the NICU can be a result of other health complications such as severe jaundice, congenital issues, disease, or birth trauma. Regardless of the reasons for a NICU stay, if a mother wishes to provide breast milk for her baby, pumping usually becomes a necessity in order to establish milk supply and provide a good foundation for long-term milk production. When a baby is unable to latch and nurse directly, expressing milk is a viable alternative.

And breast milk is, in almost all cases, exceptionally valuable for an ill or premature infant. There are critical exposure periods for breast milk, including the first days when colostrum, containing growth factors, anti-inflammatory and anti-infective properties, and of course all important nutrients, provides a vital immunity boost to an infant. A second critical period is between days fourteen to twenty-eight. Breast milk during this period has been shown to reduce a number of dangers to premature infants. While higher doses of breast milk provide increased benefits, it is important to realize that these benefits exist even if a baby is not fed breast milk exclusively.[1] Any amount of breast milk you can provide will be helping to strengthen your baby.

Having a baby in the NICU is stressful and it can feel as though you have no control over the situation — and certainly no control over your baby. While all mothers need to practice self-care and personal advocacy, it is even more important for moms with babies in the NICU. The best practices for mothers with babies in the NICU also differ slightly from mothers of full-term healthy babies. In this chapter we'll discuss the importance of self-care, the importance of good pumping habits, some techniques to help with milk production, managing and transporting your breast milk, and the inevitable question: "How can I transition my baby to breastfeeding?"

Care for Yourself So You Can Care for Your Baby

This is an important piece of advice for all new mothers, but mothers with babies in the NICU need to heed this advice the most. It's natural for mothers to turn all attention away from themselves and towards their new babies, but the added stress of hospital visits, a baby's health concerns, and financial pressures can quickly add up and become overwhelming. Mothers of preemies and babies in the NICU are more likely to have had traumatic childbirth experiences and the possibility of maternal health concerns or c-sections. Not only do babies need to heal and strengthen while they are in the NICU, but mothers need to as well. Some research has shown that a significant number of parents of babies who spent time in the NICU suffer from symptoms consistent with post-traumatic stress disorder.[2] Don't diminish your emotions and "tough it out". Self-care and understanding are extremely important during this time.

Simple practices such as sleeping when you can, eating well, and ensuring you are drinking enough water are good places to start, but they don't address the whole of your experience. You definitely need to care for your physical health, but you also need to care for your mental health. Post-partum depression is more likely to occur in mothers who experience birth trauma, breastfeeding difficulties, or other complications. It isn't really that surprising. You've just gone through an incredibly challeng-ing experience and here you are, still surrounded with the unknown and the potential for increased stress on a daily basis. This is the time to call on your support system.

Family and friends can be a physical and emotional support, assisting with many daily tasks that you don't have time for and helping you balance the additional demands, but sometimes it is difficult for people to support you when they haven't experi-enced what you are going through. For this reason, I also recommend seeking out the support of other mothers who share a similar experience. Some hospitals will offer support groups for parents of babies in the NICU. If there is a social worker on the NICU staff, speak with them and learn about the resources available to you. Use the power of the internet. There are many discussion groups and online support groups for moms. Find one that you connect with. If your NICU experience is the result of a specific health concern, look for support from those groups. It is important that you not go through this alone. Find support and accept support. Your baby has the support of all the doctors and nurses in the hospital, but you need support as well.

Pumping for your baby will empower you as a mother: you are, after all, the only one who can provide your milk for your baby. At the same time, though, pumping can be tiring and can quickly become overwhelming. It is easy to lose sight of the big picture and forget why you are pumping. A baby needs his mother—a mother who is healthy and strong. Pumping and calculating total daily volumes can easily consume your life. While breast milk is extremely valuable for a premature or ill baby, and will provide the excellent nutrition needed for growth and development, even more important is a mother who is able to be there for her child. Balance your life and your efforts. Consider carefully the options and do not be afraid to admit it is too much for you. Ask for help—demand help—and accept it when offered.

Pumps

In the case of a baby in the NICU, a hospital-grade pump is the best option. Since you do not have the benefit of nursing to establish your supply, use the best quality pump available to ensure success down the road. Once established, you may choose to change to a personal double-electric pump, but now is not the time to skimp or experiment. Mothers of preemies, especially very early preemies, may have a more difficult time establishing their supply since their breasts might not have been fully prepared for milk production and their hormone levels might not be where they would be if the baby had been born full term. It is important to be aware of this, adopt good pumping habits, and seek out the advice of a lactation consultant who has experience working with mothers of premature babies. It can sometimes just take a bit more time and consistent practice to build your milk supply, but in almost all cases it will happen.

A Good Pumping Routine

When a baby is born earlier than 34 weeks gestation, it is almost always necessary to initiate milk supply with the use of a breast pump. Babies of 34 weeks gestation and older can sometimes breastfeed from birth, although it will often be more challenging than with a full-term baby and help from a lactation consultant is strongly recommended. Start expressing early and consistently.

It is important that you begin pumping soon after delivery. Prolactin levels spike in the early hours after delivery and remain high for the first few days. Just as it is important to breastfeed early, it is important to start pumping early in order to take advantage of these high prolactin levels (you may remember that prolactin allows the initiation of lactation). Some research has shown that pumping mothers have increased volumes of milk when they begin pumping within six hours of delivery, express more than five times in a twenty-four hour period, keep a record of pumping sessions and production, and enjoy skin-to-skin contact with their babies (which we'll talk about soon).[3]

I've already discussed how to initiate supply in "Exclusively Pumping 101: The Basics", but we'll cover it briefly again here in case you only have time to read this chapter. In the early days, pumping eight to twelve times a day (including throughout the night) for about ten to fifteen minutes per session (depending on how often you are pumping) will provide you with an excellent start. During the early hours and days, frequency is really important, so the more often you can pump the better. Frequency is more important than length of sessions during this period, so extra sessions, even if they are short, will all help. Once your milk begins to increase, usually between three and five days post-partum, you should continue with at least eight sessions per 24-hour period with sessions lasting around fifteen to twenty minutes. You can stretch the time between sessions during the night so you are only waking to pump once between the hours of 1 a.m. and 5 a.m. and getting a few more hours of sleep; however, it is a good idea at this stage not to go much more than five hours without pumping at night and no more than three hours during the day. Frequency of stimulation is extremely important, so while pumping every two hours during the day may seem extreme it will help to establish a strong supply not just in the early weeks but for the months ahead. In general, you want to maintain around the same total number of minutes pumping per day regardless of how often you are pumping.[4] 120 minutes per day is a good guide for pumping.

When you are pumping, it is beneficial to use an expressing pattern that is as similar to a breastfeeding baby as possible; although you haven't yet become conditioned to your baby's nursing pattern, using a this type of pattern will help you initiate a stronger let-down response. Babies don't suck at the same rate or strength throughout a nursing session. Instead, they begin with fast, light suckles. This continues until the milk ejection response. At this point, a baby will begin to take deeper, slower draws at the breast until the flow slows at which time the baby will return to the lighter, more frequent suckling if she is still hungry. While some breast pumps offer a similar pattern built into them, it isn't necessary to get a pump that does this for you. Instead, as long as you have a pump that allows you to adjust the cycling speed (the speed of the suck and release) and the suction level, you'll be able to make these adjustments based on your body's response to the pump. And speaking of your body, don't forget an important part of your body that can greatly increase your success exclusively pumping: your hands.

Let Your Hands Work for You

In the first few days following the birth of your baby, your milk supply will be low but colostrum is being produced and is the perfect first food for your baby. Colostrum can be difficult to express because it is thick and sticky. Often it will get caught in the pump flanges and valves. You can use a syringe to collect as much colostrum as possible from the pump flanges and bottle, but there is another way to collect colostrum: hand expression. Being able to hand express can be a "handy" skill to have, but it can also markedly increase your milk supply. Aside from using hand expression techniques to collect colostrum, combining hand expression with the use of a breast pump and "hands-on pumping" techniques—both breast massage and breast compressions—have been shown to increase a pre-term mother's milk supply.[5]

Hand expression is quite simple once you get the hang of it, but it is something that is best seen. For this reason, I encourage you to view an excellent video produced by Dr. Jane Morton and the Stanford School of Medicine. The video, which is just over seven minutes in length, provides clear information on how to use your hands to express milk.[6]

In addition to hand expression, you can use your hands while you use the breast pump. These hands-on techniques will help remove more milk and ultimately cut down on the length of time you need to pump in order to remove milk. The two different techniques to learn, and use, are breast compressions and breast massage.

Breast compressions are often used by breastfeeding mothers, and the concept is the same. When you are experiencing a let-down, place the thumb on one side of the breast and the fingers on the other, close to the chest wall. Once your fingers are in place, compress the breast with your fingers firmly but not to the point of pain or discomfort. Hold the pressure until the flow of milk slows or the spot feels softer. You can then move your fingers to a different position on the breast and apply pressure again. Keep the pressure closer to the chest wall than the areola. Applying pressure too close to the areola can actually reduce milk flow by blocking the milk ducts.

Breast massage can also be used along with compressions. To massage the breasts, apply firm but gentle massage in circular motions all around the breast. Massage can be particularly useful if there are ducts that aren't draining well or hard spots in the breast. Massage can be done before you pump or while you are pumping. To make it easier to use both massage and compressions while you pump, you might consider wearing a hands-free pumping bra.

Another benefit of using these hands-on techniques in conjunction with pumping is the increase of fat that is released into the milk. Research has shown that mothers who combine the use of massage and compression and manual expression have high levels of fat and calorically dense milk.[7] This is particularly important for preemies—who need every calorie they can get.

One study conducted by Dr. Jane Morton looked specifically at combining pumping with hands-on pumping techniques and hand expression. Using hospital-grade pumps, mothers double-pumped eight times a day for fifteen minutes per session for the first three days. They also hand expressed colostrum as frequently as possible during this time. Once their milk volumes began to increase (mature milk began), they were instructed to pump eight times a day until they were only expressing drops. After being discharged, the mothers were followed at the hospital and taught hands-on pumping techniques. Once milk flow stopped, they stopped pumping, massaged their breasts for a short period, and then attempted to remove any remaining milk using either the breast pump or manual expression. For all study participants, the mean volume of milk expressed rose to

820 mL/day by week eight, but for women who had hand expressed more than five times during the first three days post-partum their mean volume was 955 mL/day. What's even more compelling is that daily volumes for the three days prior to hands-on pumping techniques being taught were compared to daily volumes at eight weeks and an increase of 48% was seen. 92.9% of the mothers had an increase in milk production. Certainly, hands-on pumping is the way to go.

Kangaroo Care

Skin-to-skin contact with your baby is a wonderful way to connect and bond, but it also is beneficial to your milk supply. When used with preemies, skin-to-skin contact is known as kangaroo mother care or KMC. Time spent skin-to-skin has been shown to raise prolactin levels in the mother, which in turn helps to boost milk production. The mother's warmth and regular breathing help the baby maintain body temperature and regulate respiration. Amid all the stress of the NICU, KMC can be a time to relax and get to know your baby. Not only is KMC an important part of your baby's care, it has also been shown to change a mother's perception of her child.[8, 9]

At its simplest, KMC involves sitting in a reclined position with your baby on your chest, skin-to-skin, with a wrap or blanket covering both you and your baby—there are even shirts and wraps made specifically for KMC. While many NICUs will not allow KMC until a baby is considered stable, Dr. Nils Berg-man's research suggests that the best place for a premature baby is with the mother, practising KMC, and that low birth weight infants placed with the mother in the first six hours following birth stabilized more quickly than infants placed in incubators.[10] If your hospital does not suggest kangaroo mother care, ask for it. It's an incredible time of relaxation and snuggles that you will always cherish.

Milk Management and Storage

Every pumping mom needs to deal with milk management and storage, but mothers who are pumping for babies in the NICU also have the added requirement of transporting breast milk to the hospital. The NICU should provide guidelines for handling breast milk for a preemie. Due to a premature baby's more fragile state of health, it is important to be particularly aware of possible contamination of breast milk and safe handling practices. Preemies' immune systems will not function as well as those of full-term babies and they are at higher risk of complications such as necrotizing enterocolitis. Your milk is incredibly beneficial in protecting against possible infection and complications, but at the same time you don't want to introduce any infection through your milk.

In terms of your pump and pump kit (flanges and other removable parts), it is important to keep everything as clean as possible. Sterilization of your pump kit is something that should be done regularly. If you are pumping in the hospital, I would recommend sterilizing after every pumping session. While this is a great deal of added work, the hospital environment is not sterile and there are many germs and bacteria in hospitals. When you are at home, you are okay to sterilize once a day. Sterilization can be done in a pot of boiling water for 5-10 minutes (follow the pump kit manufacturer's guidelines if given) or you can use a steam sterilizer. Some dishwashers will also bring the temperature to a sufficient level to sterilize. Aside from the pump kit, it is good practice to wipe down the pump before you use it. You can use premoistened antibacterial wipes or even a baby wipe in a pinch. And before you do anything, be sure to wash your hands well. Collection bottles should be sterile and can be sterilized along with your pump kit.

Check with your hospital to see if they have a preference for storage bottles. When I was pumping, the NICU provided bags of small orange-lidded specimen bottles. It is important to use small containers, since your preemie will only be taking small amounts of milk at first and larger containers may mean that some milk is not used before it needs to be discarded. One thing that is absolutely critical is that your milk be labelled. Obviously it is important that *your* milk is given to *your* baby, so labelling should be done according to the hospital's policies. Most NICUs will require you to label the milk with your name, the date it was expressed, your baby's name, and possibly an identifying number or code.

You'll also need to figure out a system for transporting milk to the hospital. When you pump at the hospital you can leave that milk with your baby. The nurses will likely use the fresh milk as much as possible, but milk that is not used immediately may be placed in the refrigerator or in a freezer in the NICU. Check to see how much milk your baby needs and how much milk the NICU would like you to leave with them. A cooler bag and some cold packs are all you need to transport milk from your home to the hospital. Milk—either refrigerated or frozen—will do fine in a cooler bag for a few hours.

Expressing for a preemie can be both a rewarding and isolating experience. Often it feels like the only thing you can do for your baby is to provide your milk. This can be immensely empowering and satisfying, as well as disappointing and painful. You are doing what no one else can, but as a mother we want more. Know that what you are doing is incredibly important, but do seek out other opportunities to be involved in your baby's care. Feed her when possible, ask to be present for baths and to help when possible, take responsibility for oral care when you're at the hospital, and ask questions about your baby's progress and care. Your presence and love are extremely valuable. You are your baby's mother and you have an important role in your baby's care.

Transitioning to Breastfeeding

A lengthy discussion on how to transition a premature baby to exclusive breastfeeding is beyond the scope of this book; however, I wanted to provide a few resources and words of advice to assist you if your desire is to ultimately breastfeed your baby. Regardless of the reasons for your baby's NICU stay, if you are unable to breastfeed from birth then pumping becomes extremely important. Initiating a good milk supply will give you options down the road. A good milk supply will make it easier for your baby to transition to the breast, since milk flow will be strong. So as paradoxical as it may seem, one of the first things you need to do to transition to breastfeeding is ensure you are pumping and establishing your milk supply.

Transitioning from exclusively pumping to exclusively breastfeeding can require a leap of faith. When pumping and feeding expressed breast milk, it is easy to feel as though you have some control of the process. You control when you pump and you can see how much your baby is eating. When it comes to breastfeeding, you don't have the same sense of control. But remember that this is how it is supposed to be. One of the wonderful things about breastfeeding is not having to measure and prepare and monitor. It is important that you're prepared to let go of that control and to empower yourself with knowledge of what breastfeeding looks like.

How you approach breastfeeding can make a big difference, especially if you've had a bit of a rocky start. Choose an approach to breastfeeding that is relaxing and unhurried. Two such approaches are baby-led latching, championed by Christina Smillie, and biological nurturing, developed by Suzanne Colson. The subtitle of Suzanne Colson's website is "laid back breastfeeding" and Colson's work and ideas are based on that idea in both a literal and figurative sense. Breastfeeding should most definitely be "laid back" in the sense that it shouldn't be stressful and should seamlessly fit into your daily life. Breastfeeding positions can also be laid back, both in attitude and practice.

Colson describes biological nurturing (BN) in this way:

> BN is laid back breastfeeding: mothers neither sit upright nor do they lie on their sides or flat on their backs. Instead, they are in comfortable semi-reclined positions where every part of their body is supported, especially their shoulders and neck. Then they lay their babies on top of their bodies so that baby's head is somewhere near the breast. In other words mothers make the breast available. Babies lie prone or on their tummies but their bodies are not flat but tilted up.[11]

On her website, Biological Nurturing, Colson presents these basic beliefs about breastfeeding:

- Mothers and babies are versatile feeders. There is not one way to breastfeed.
- A baby does not need to be awake to latch on and feed.
- Babies often self-attach; mothers can help them do this.
- Babies often have reflex movements called cues indicating they are ready to feed whilst asleep.
- Looking for baby reflex feeding cues helps mothers to get to know their babies sooner. This increases confidence.
- Crying and hunger cues are late feeding indicators often making latching difficult. Getting started with breastfeeding is about releasing baby feeding reflexes as stimulants, helping ba-

bies find the breast, latch on and feed... not about interest.

- The breastfeeding position the baby uses often mimics the baby in the womb.
- There is no right or wrong breastfeeding position. The right position is the one that works.
- Babies do not always feed for hunger; "non nutritive sucking" is hugely beneficial to increase your milk and satisfy your baby's needs.[12]

Breastfeeding should be a time of relaxation for both mom and baby, but all too often new mothers are stressed and anxious about breastfeeding their newborns. Breastfeeding supporters often show new moms very specific breastfeeding positions or even physically handle mom and baby to try to force a latch. Having had this experience myself when my son was still in the NICU, I know how humiliating and stressful this can be, and I've heard from many women who have had similar experiences and who talk of how violated and uncomfortable they felt with such aggressive breastfeeding support—regardless of how well-meaning it may have been.

Suzanne Colson approaches breastfeeding from a perspective of calm and relaxation. Not only is this the approach for the actual act of breastfeeding, but for the way that breastfeeding fits into your life. Breastfeeding should be easy; it should fit easily into your life. While it is true that many women today have life situations that take them outside of the home during the day and do not allow for full-time breastfeeding, even in these cases breastfeeding when you are with your child can be an easy, stress-reducing way of mothering, bonding with, and nurturing your baby.

I strongly encourage you to visit Suzanne Colson's website, www.biologicalnurturing.com, and learn more about her ideas and suggestions for breastfeeding. Her article, "A non-prescriptive recipe for breastfeeding", available on her website, is a great introduction to the idea of biological nurturing. She has also published a book called *An Introduction to Biological Nurturing*. If you have an interest in using the method with your baby, you might consider purchasing a copy or asking for it at your local library.

Christina Smillie has extensively researched newborns' breastfeeding abilities and her approach, based on this research, is commonly referred to as baby-led latching. Dr. Smillie recognizes that babies have a sequence of behaviours that lead them to latching. When this sequence is followed, latching becomes easier and less stressful for both mom and baby.

Babies are born with reflexes that assist them in breastfeeding. These reflexes include the following:

- Stepping and crawling, which help a baby get to the breast.
- Searching, rooting, sight, and smell, which help a baby find the breast.
- Rooting and opening the mouth, helping a baby attach to the breast.
- Sucking, which is stimulated when a baby feels the nipple in the mouth.

Skin-to-skin contact on the mother's chest stimulates a baby's sense of smell and touch, which initiates feeding behaviours. A calm, attentive state—for both mother and baby—assists in feeding behaviours and helps the newborn find the breast and successfully breastfeed. It is important to find a position in which you are comfortable (just as Suzanne Colson suggests). A relaxed mom is just as important as a relaxed baby.

The following is a brief overview of baby-led latching:

- Place baby in a vertical position between your breasts, skin-to-skin. Your baby can be in a diaper. You should be in a somewhat reclined position.
- Support your baby's neck and shoulders but not the head. A baby has a reflex to push back on anything holding its head.
- Support your baby's bottom as well. You can use the crook of your arm to support your baby's rump and legs. Your baby needs to feel safe and secure.
- Follow your baby's lead: if baby wants to sleep, sleep is okay. Allow your baby to set the pace. Your job is to keep your baby calm.
- When your baby gets hungry, she will start to search for the breast by bobbing her head around. Support the baby's neck and shoulders as the baby moves towards the breast but allow free head movement.
- Support your baby's bottom with the other hand and keep your baby's tummy tight to your chest. Do not allow the legs to flail around. Help your baby feel secure.
- If necessary, help your baby line up with the nipple: nose to nipple and chin in close contact with the breast. Your baby will likely nuzzle, lick, and taste before actually latching. Be patient and allow your baby to figure it all out.
- Calm and talk to your baby throughout. If your baby is anxious, soothe him by talking gently or making shhhhing sounds. If necessary, you may

need to remove your baby from your chest and swaddle and soothe him before returning him skin-to-skin.

- Do not try to force your baby to the breast. Only offer the breast when your baby is calm. Pay attention to early feeding cues and keep your newborn skin-to-skin as much as possible to allow frequent feeding at the baby's pace.
- If your baby has had difficulty establishing breastfeeding or has refused to latch, baby-led latching can be a gentle way to encourage breast-feeding.[13]

There is a significant amount of information on the internet about baby-led latching including numerous videos. What is most important with this approach is the respect for the biological process and the understanding that babies are born with a great many skills to assist them to breastfeed successfully. Trusting our babies and allowing them to follow their own instincts can go a long way to establishing a strong breastfeeding relationship.

Chapter 11

Relationships
(With a Little Help from Your Friends)

Becoming a mother alters your life in ways you can't imagine before having kids. Changes in your relationships with family, friends, your spouse, and older children are almost inevitable. These changes are often positive and serve to build deeper, stronger relationships, but sometimes achieving a stronger relationship can mean working through new challenges and overcoming new obstacles. The good news is that with planning and understanding everything can work out, resulting in a stronger relationship between you and the important people in your life. While exclusively pumping doesn't cause problems that are wholly unfamiliar to other moms, still, as with any unique situation, it may require creative or specially tailored solutions.

A good place to start is to be as open with your family and friends as possible and allow them to understand your decision to pump. Exclusively pumping is something that you as a mother need to adjust to, particularly if your desire was to breastfeed your baby, but it is equally important to recognize that your family and friends may need to adjust to it as well. When you consider the additional time commitment that is required by pumping moms you can quickly begin to see how this feeding option will influence the lives of those you love.

This chapter will offer some suggestions for building a relationship with your new baby while maintaining a strong relationship with your older children, family, friends, and spouse. The suggestions are by no means an exhaustive list but will perhaps start you thinking about how your entire support circle is affected by your decision to exclusively pump and ways in which they can learn to support you. We'll also consider ways you can spend quality time with your friends and family — and maybe even add in a little bit of "me" time.

Building a Strong Bond with Your New Baby

Earlier in the chapter on lactation and breast milk composition, the role and importance of oxytocin was discussed. Oxytocin, you'll remember, is responsible for a number of things including contractions during labour and the milk ejection response. One of the most interesting roles of oxytocin, however, is its role in love and bonding. Oxytocin helps to create social bonds between people and is released during activities such as sex, when it is important to bond with your partner; breastfeeding, when it is important for mother and baby to bond; and even during mealtime, when those sharing a meal become a single unit and bond around common experience. While a pumping mom and her baby will not benefit from the release of oxytocin during breastfeeding, this isn't to say that bonding won't happen.

Unfortunately, sometimes a woman who exclusively pumps is told by others that she is doing her baby a disservice by not breastfeeding and that she will not build a strong bond with her baby because she is not breastfeeding. Breastfeeding does provide an excellent opportunity for mother and baby to bond, but it is by no means the only way a mother and baby bond. Please remember that mothering is about far more than the way we feed our babies and that bonding goes well beyond food. The following are some suggestions for building a strong bond with your new baby:

- Oxytocin peaks during the first hours after your baby's birth. Share some quiet one-on-one time with your baby after delivery. Consider putting off all unnecessary practices such as weighing and cleaning your baby, and instead snuggle with your new baby on your chest, taking in the moment and enjoying the culmination of the last nine months. If kept skin-to-skin, your baby will stay warm under a blanket. Oxytocin floods the brain with a wash of good feelings and when your baby is the object of your attention, the bond between you will strengthen.
- Make time for your new baby. Leave other things such as the dishes or vacuuming when possible. Go for a walk, snuggle for a nap, go shopping together, lay on the floor and play: it doesn't matter what you're doing, but ensure that you don't put so much of yourself into other activities that you feel you are missing out on getting to know, and spend time with, your baby.
- Lots of skin-to-skin contact with your baby, especially in the early days, can help to establish a strong bond and will also aid in milk production. Take a break in the afternoon and lie down with your baby on your chest. Not only will you enjoy the closeness, but your baby will also benefit

from your warmth and the connection he will have to your breathing and heart beat.

- Do not "bottle prop", merely propping the bottle in the baby's mouth while your attention is on other things or other people. Turn off the television when feeding your baby. Use the time to gaze at him, sing, talk, smile, laugh, and enjoy those early, squishy newborn days. This may not always be a realistic—I know that sometimes other things do demand your attention when feeding your baby—but be conscious of how you are interacting with your child when bottle feeding.

- Consider wearing your baby in a sling, wrap, mei tai, or other type of carrier. Wearing your baby not only frees you up to do other things while still meeting the needs of your child, but it also meets your baby's need for physical contact, security, stimulation, and movement. Babies worn in a carrier often cry less than babies not worn. The baby's close proximity to you will also assist in maintaining body temperature and regulating respiration and heart rate.

- Pumping hands-free can allow you to play with your baby while pumping. Using a hands-free pumping bra will give you the freedom to sit on the floor, read a book to your baby, or play with your baby, all while getting in your daily pumping sessions.

- Recognize that you are providing nourishment for your baby. While it may take some time away from her, it is providing a lot as well. It is a bal-

ancing act that will take you a little time to get
used to. Be patient and be kind to yourself.

Your Relationship With Other Children

A new baby can be an enormous adjustment for older siblings.
While not always the case, some older siblings will go through a
period of jealousy or anger at losing out on the status he or she
might have enjoyed. For some children this rivalry never seems
to end! Suddenly, there is a new baby that must fit into their
world, a new baby for which *they* must make accommodations.
You will no doubt have considered ways to make this adjustment easier on your children.

When you start to exclusively pump, you are now adding
another element of change into your child's life. You may not
have as much time to spend with your older child and you may
find that you are staying closer to home for a few weeks when
you are frequently pumping. This can be a challenging adjustment for a young child that is used to getting out of the house for
activities and who has had free access to mom whenever it was
desired. Here are a few ideas to help older children adjust to all
the new things happening in your home and ways to maintain a
strong relationship with them while you are pumping:

- Depending on their age, explain to them what
  you are doing and why you are doing it. Use language that they can understand—don't get too
  technical. Explain that mommy's milk is the best
  food for babies and you need to pump to provide
  the baby milk. There are some great books available about breastfeeding and breast milk. You
  might consider searching for one or two and
  making it part of your regular book rotation.[1]

- Explain how you fed them and why you are feeding the new baby this way. This is a wonderful opportunity to focus the attention on your older child. They will learn that you loved and cared for them when they were little just as you are caring for your new baby. Having this discussion also sets the stage for later discussions about babies, pregnancy, and all the fascinating discussions that young children want to have. Why not start paving the "birds and bees" path now?

- Include your older child in your daily routine. Give them special tasks such as turning on the pump, bringing you things you might need while you are pumping, or watching the baby while you pump. Let them be an important element of your success. Tasks will vary depending on the age of your child, but all children love to be useful and needed.

- Consider your time pumping as an opportunity to spend time with older children. For example, if your baby is sleeping and doesn't require your attention when you pump, give this time to your older child: read a story, sing songs, or play games such as "I Spy" or "Simon Says" that don't require too much participation on your part.

- Make pumping time a special time for your older child. Have a basket of toys that your child gets to play with only when you pump; find a special movie that gets turned on when the pump turns on; or if your child is a bit older, perhaps make pumping time video game time. This will help make the time something to look forward to.

If your older child is still quite young and unable to understand what you are doing or unable to be on his own while you pump, recognize that he may see the pump and the new baby as something that has taken his mother away. Be prepared to spend some one-on-one time with your child and recognize that new behaviours may simply be a reaction to this change. Be patient and understanding. Try not to see your older children as another obstacle to pumping. It might prove more challenging with another child in the house, but working together and learning to see the opportunities will help you build a special relationship.

Your Relationship with Friends and Family

Hopefully, most of your friends and family will be supportive of your decision to exclusively pump. However, some will not understand why you don't just breastfeed and some won't understand why you don't just feed formula—you can never win! Both opinions can be frustrating and difficult to tolerate, especially if you are already under stress.

For those people who want you to feed formula, simply explain the benefits of breast milk and explain how you want to provide the very best for your baby. Suggest that they too, no doubt, want the best for your child and you are thankful that now, having this information, they will support your decision. Do not give them the option to continue with their former position. Often comments such as theirs are not so much unsupportive of your decision to pump as they are showing concern for you and the amount of time and effort they see you putting into expressing milk for your baby.

Sometimes people also fall victim to the overwhelming advertising from formula companies that often claim formula to be "close to mother's milk." People need to be educated about breast milk and infant formula. Many older adults fed their children formula as babies and may have some lingering grief or regret over their experiences. It is often hard to look beyond your own situation, but by doing so you can often see where others are coming from.

It is often more difficult to sway the opinions of those who believe you should be breastfeeding. Some simply don't understand why you would "choose" to pump even though for many women it is not a choice they wanted to make. People often don't recognize the exclusively pumping mother as having made a better choice than feeding formula. And some critics see exclusively pumping as second rate to breastfeeding and may say you are doing your baby a disservice—or worse, harming your baby. They may feel that every woman can breastfeed if she truly wants to breastfeed. This is simply not true, and while I'd love to be able to tell you to ignore those people and move on, I realize that sometimes these hurtful comments can come from those you love and those who should be supporting you. What people like this tend to forget is that breastfeeding is a biological activity but it must be socially supported. Our society is doing a crummy job of supporting breastfeeding moms and often breastfeeding support is lacking, the birth process is often counter to successful breastfeeding, and in many countries breastfeeding is often made difficult due to the lack of maternity leave and the lack of recognition for a mother's rights and needs in public places and the workplace.

Regardless of a person's stance, all you can do is explain your position: why you are not breastfeeding and why you chose to exclusively pump instead of feed formula. Be understanding of how they may feel threatened by your dedication and determination, especially if they fed formula to their baby. Recognize most people's intentions are good. They may not realize how emotional it can be for you right now. If you know the person well and want them to support you through the experience, share your emotions. Don't be afraid to tell them that you are scared, grieving, lost, hopeful, relieved, or however you may be feeling. By sharing your emotions, those around you will be able to understand your experience better and reframe their opinions to get onside with you.

Here are a few thoughts on maintaining a strong relationship with friends and family:

- Explain that a happy, healthy baby makes you happy and healthy and also that their support and friendship will make it easier for you to continue.
- Avoid, as much as possible, those people who continue to be negative or outwardly unsupportive of your decision — it can be easy to give in to the will of others. While cutting people out can be hard, sometimes it is necessary. So many women tend to be pleasers; we will bend over backwards to keep others happy while all the while being miserable ourselves. Now is the time to focus on you and your baby. You are not being selfish to expect support from those around you. If they can't give it, or at least keep quiet about their reservations, then it is okay to limit their influence in your life.
- Stay focused on your goals and let those around you know what your goals are so they can help you to achieve them. You don't need to go it alone, so share your goals — and your fears — and allow those around you to provide support.
- Become as mobile as possible. Some people may simply wish they could see more of you and feel that exclusively pumping is taking away your ability to visit them or do things with them.

Make it clear that you are happy to visit, but you'll come with your pump and need to pump while you are there. This isn't too much to ask for, is it? Having other people in the house can be extremely helpful. They can watch the baby and allow you time to take care of yourself and perhaps even get a bit of a break. You might prefer people come to your house—and that can be a great option—but don't overlook the benefits of visiting someone else's house.

- Build new support systems when needed. Reach out into your community for new mothers' programs, play groups, church groups, or La Leche League meetings. Don't overlook online communities as well. With a little bit of searching, you'll be able to find other women who are experiencing many of the same things you are and who are eager to both receive and extend support. Some of your best friends may be found online.

Your Relationship with Your Spouse

Simply adding a new baby into your life can be enough to turn your relationship with your spouse upside down. Regardless of whether this is your first baby or not, adding a new life into your world takes some adjustment. Many men find it difficult to fit into the baby's world and see mothers as the ones who know everything: moms just naturally know what to do and what's going on, right? It is important to involve your spouse as much as possible in the baby's daily activities, both for his benefit, the baby's benefit, and your own benefit.

Most spouses simply want their wives to be okay and seeing her stressed and exhausted and possibly in pain from a poor breastfeeding experience or pumping can be very concerning for them. This concern can sometimes manifest itself as being unsupportive of pumping. They may suggest a switch to formula not because they are contrary or do not want the baby to receive breast milk, but because they see how difficult it is for their wives. While some husbands are unsupportive, most are incredibly supportive and simply want you to be okay. Men naturally want to be able to fix things, so you might need to ask your husband *not* to fix the problem but instead to simply listen to you and understand.

Share with your spouse the value of feeding breast milk for both you and your baby. Enlist him to help educate family and friends; a united front can go a long way in swaying unsupportive family members. Also, tell your spouse how you feel about not breastfeeding. Often men find it difficult to relate to a new mother's emotions and do not realize how emotional the act of breastfeeding can be. Help him to understand this as best you can. Explain to him how his unwavering support is absolutely necessary for you to be successful exclusively pumping.

Suggest ways your spouse can support you and make things easier:

- Cleaning bottles and your pump kit
- Caring for your older children
- Bathing the baby
- Feeding the baby
- Allowing you to relax and perhaps giving a back rub or foot rub
- Not mentioning weaning or feeding formula unless you have introduced the subject
- Being flexible and understanding your time is not as free as it once was
- Taking care of the household chores that you are unable to do easily such as outside work, grocery

shopping, banking, and cooking the occasional dinner
- And whatever else you feel would support your ability to be successful exclusively pumping!

Some other things to consider:

- Talk to your spouse when you are pumping. Often this might be the only uninterrupted one-on-one time you will get during a day.
- Understand that you may feel differently about your body after having a baby as well as while you are pumping. Share this with your spouse.
- Take advantage of people offering to babysit in order to spend some time with your spouse.
- Don't place expectations on your relationship. Understand it will evolve and change. Be flexible and patient and, most of all, have a sense of humour!
- Find support with other couples and mothers and talk with them about changes in their relationships.
- Lactation changes hormone levels in your body which can affect you in many ways. You may have a reduced sex drive and may experience vaginal dryness. These may not normalize until after you have weaned. You may want to speak to your doctor if they are particularly troublesome.

Don't Ignore Your Own Needs

Amidst all the busyness of your day, it can be easy to forget about yourself or to push your needs to the bottom of the to-do list. But caring for yourself must be given priority. As mothers, we are most effective if we are healthy, happy, and feeling balanced. Give yourself time after the birth of your baby to adjust to all the changes, both in your life and your body. No matter how you feed your baby, adjusting to motherhood takes time. With the excitement of bringing home your new baby, you also are experiencing a wide range of emotions. Hormones are on a roller coaster ride, and you are often expected to keep it all together and get on with the work of being a new mom. But is this really a fair expectation? Some cultures allow new mothers a "babymoon", allowing them to rest for several weeks, healing from childbirth, and bonding with their babies.

Think about what makes you happy, what centres you, and what refills you when you're feeling run down or de-energized. Do you enjoy taking a relaxing bath, getting out with friends, an invigorating walk? Take the time to do these things. Even a short twenty minutes with the bathroom door locked to shower or soak in the tub can make you feel like a new woman. Seek out whatever makes you feel energized or relaxed and make time for it in your schedule.

Nutrition is also an important part of self-care. As life gets busy, what we eat often becomes a matter of convenience and speed, but in the end this just contributes to loss of energy and becoming run down. Try to keep healthy snacks stocked in your fridge and pantry. Buy cut up veggies or baby carrots. Have nuts or healthy trail mix handy. When you cook, think big and make double batches when possible; freeze the extra, giving you an easy meal on those days when time is at a premium. Cook big pots of soup, stew, or chili—again, easy to freeze and nutritious. Don't be afraid to ask friends, family, or your church to help you by making casseroles and other freezable foods. You might even consider getting together with some friends and making big batches of food to share.

Joining forces with other moms is also a great way to ease the daily tasks while you are at home. The extra hands make it easier for you to get chores done in the house knowing that someone else is there to help with your baby. The camaraderie can also be an important benefit for all mothers, regardless of how you're feeding your baby.

Sleep is often in short supply when you are a new parent — well, perhaps for all parents regardless of how old your child is. Mothers are often encouraged to "sleep when your baby sleeps", but, for moms who are exclusively pumping, this usually becomes prime pumping time. Still, sleep is important and you need to balance it. Since others can feed your baby, you may be able to sneak in some extra snooze time every once in awhile. If your spouse can take the night feedings, then you'll only need to pump during the night and this will allow you to get back to bed sooner than if you were pumping and feeding your baby at night. As you continue pumping, you'll eventually be able to extend your length of sleep at night. In the meantime, get it where and when you can, and take some solace in the fact that around the world there are millions of other sleep deprived parents who are going through the same thing.

Finally, be aware of how you are feeling emotionally. Post-partum depression is real and it can be treated. Women who have had traumatic birth experiences or breastfeeding challenges are at a higher risk for post-partum depression. If you feel sad, low, anxious, moody, or find you can't sleep, you may have what is commonly referred to as "the baby blues", but if they continue for more than two weeks and include a loss of appetite, difficulty bonding with your baby, withdrawal from your family and friends, or thoughts of harming yourself or your baby, it is absolutely vital that you reach out and talk to someone as soon as possible as you may be experiencing post-partum depression.

Taking care of yourself and your baby sometimes means you need to allow others to take care of you.

Chapter 12

You Can Do It!
Overcoming Challenges

As much as we hope things will always go smoothly in life, this just isn't always the case. There are a number of challenges that you might experience when exclusively pumping and being prepared for them and knowing how to handle them will make it all that much easier to resolve the problem and move on. As with many things in life, time will often resolve the problems you encounter; however, when you are in the middle of the situation, it is often difficult to remove yourself from the present and see things in perspective. Remember that you will be pumping for only a short time when you balance it out in terms of your life or your child's life. While it may not seem possible, time will pass and you will move with it. Each pumping session will take you closer to your goal. The first couple months of your new baby's life will move at a snail's pace and every problem you encounter will be magnified as you become accustomed to your new life. With any difficulty you encounter, recognize that it will usually pass with time and that things will soon settle into a comfortable routine. Very few challenges are insurmountable, yet some require a little extra time and effort. This chapter is intended to help you through the challenges you may encounter, giving you information to enable you to persevere and conquer any problem you may experience.

Delayed Lactogenesis II

There are a number of reasons why lactogenesis II might be delayed. Normally, a new mother's milk supply will begin to increase within about 3-5 days after delivery. Women who have other children will find their milk increases earlier than first-time mothers. Generally it is just a matter of frequent and consistent stimulation of the breasts, nipples, and areolas, and lactogenesis II will begin as it should. However, there are a number of factors that can cause delayed lactogenesis II. You can't always control these causes, but recognizing them will help you to plan your next steps and recognize when you may require additional support from a lactation consultant:

- Certain labour interventions or health conditions (e.g. diabetes, PCOS) can affect the onset of lactogenesis II; even smoking and obesity can reduce prolactin levels and have an impact on milk supply. C-sections, large intake of IV fluids, and premature deliveries can cause delays in milk production.
- The first thing is to feed the baby. You can feed any colostrum you are able to pump, but if your milk supply hasn't increased in the first couple of days, there is nothing wrong with using formula to feed your baby.
- Follow a frequent pumping schedule, even if you don't see any increase. Pumping every 2 hours

around the clock for about 10-12 minutes is your best strategy. Combining the use of a pump with hand expression is also good practice.

- Be persistent and patient. Supply will usually increase by 7-10 days post-partum.
- If supply does not increase, seek the advice of a lactation professional and return to your doctor for an examination. Although not common, retained placenta can prevent lactogenesis II. Also, other concerns such as hypoplastic breasts (insufficient glandular tissue) and previous breast surgery should be considered.

Sore Nipples and Breast Pain

Not all women who exclusively pump will be faced with nipple soreness or breast pain. While breast and nipple pain can sometimes lead a woman to consider weaning, it shouldn't ever be necessary. It is important to understand the many reasons you may experience soreness and head the problem off before it begins, or at least resolve the problem as quickly as possible.

The following are some common reasons you may experience soreness when pumping.

Engorgement

Engorgement is a common experience among new mothers, but it doesn't need to be. Engorgement happens when milk production increases and milk removal does not keep pace with production. The result is breasts that are overly full, hard, uncomfortable, and sometimes milk expression becomes difficult. Engorgement should be taken seriously, as it can lead to blocked ducts and mastitis if milk is not removed. While engorgement is most common in the early post-partum period when lactation is still controlled primarily by hormones and production is not yet stable, you can still experience engorgement weeks or months in. Those extra hours of sleep feel great, but "ouch", the full, hard breasts don't feel so great when you wake up! If you experience engorgement, follow these suggestions to relieve discomfort and prevent additional problems:

- Ensure your breast pump is appropriate for exclusively pumping and that it is working effectively.
- Pump frequently and empty breasts as much as possible.
- You can use ibuprofen or acetaminophen for discomfort.
- Use cold packs in between pumping sessions and warm, moist compresses just prior to pumping (do not use warm for more than a few minutes).
- For an effective cold pack, pour some water in a newborn disposable diaper. Shape the diaper into a u-shape and put it in the freezer to get cold. Use a cloth or towel between the diaper and breast.
- Use massage both prior to and during your pumping session.
- Use breast compressions while pumping. Firm, consistent pressure can assist in releasing ducts and removing milk (see page 128 for more info).
- Cabbage leaves have been anecdotally reported as being helpful. Use cold, crushed green cabbage leaves and place around your breasts in your bra (not on the nipple as there is a small risk of listeria) and leave until wilted. Do not overuse though as they also have been reported to reduce milk supply if used for too long.

- Wear a supportive bra 24 hours a day but do not wear underwire bras or anything that is too constricting.
- Engorgement will normally subside within 12-48 hours if properly treated.

Yeast Infection

Yeast infections, or thrush, are fairly common in breastfeeding women and unfortunately exclusively pumping mothers are not immune either. A yeast infection is characterized by a burning pain, deep tissue pain if the yeast is also in the breast ducts, redness and shininess of the nipple, itchiness, and the possibility of yeast infection in your baby's mouth or diaper area. Receiving antibiotics during labour can increase the chances of a yeast overgrowth as can a general tendency towards yeast infections.

Yeast is naturally occurring in our bodies and a yeast infection is better thought of as a yeast overgrowth. The problem is systemic, not local, and in order to treat yeast overgrowth you need to treat the whole body, not just the breast. Therefore, try to reduce your intake of sugars and simple carbohydrates as well as improve your intestinal flora by taking probiotic supplements. You can also increase your intake of fermented foods such as yogurt, kefir, and sauerkraut, all which encourage healthy gut flora. A healthy diet, strong immune system, and healthy digestive tract are vital to keeping a yeast overgrowth at bay.

If you suspect your baby may have thrush, look for white patches in your baby's mouth that do not wash off. Soreness and redness in the mouth and throat caused by the yeast can sometimes cause a baby to refuse to eat. In the diaper area, yeast will show as a red diaper rash, usually in small circles or spots and will show no improvement with the use of a diaper cream. If you think your baby has thrush, see your baby's doctor to receive treatment. Many doctors will recommend a baby be treated for thrush if the mother has been diagnosed with it and the baby is being breastfed. However, there is no evidence to suggest that expressed breast milk from a mother with thrush cannot be fed to the baby.[1]

If you develop what you think is a yeast infection, you might consider a visit to your doctor in order to develop a treatment plan. Depending on the severity of the infection, you may need to start on oral medications. However, prescription treatment is not always necessary and natural remedies and lifestyle changes can often resolve the overgrowth. Coconut oil has antifungal, antibacterial, and anti-inflammatory properties and may be considered as a treatment against yeast. Use a good quality cold-pressed, extra-virgin coconut oil and massage a small amount onto the breast and nipple area after pumping. You might also consider using it on your baby's diaper area if your baby is showing signs of thrush.[2]

It is also important to prevent re-infecting yourself with the materials that come in contact with your breasts. Yeast is particularly resilient and it may take some effort to rid your system of the overgrowth. Be sure to do the following:

- Change your breast pads frequently if you are using them.
- Wash your bras frequently in hot water.
- Wash your bath towel in hot water after every use.
- Sterilize your pump kit after every use.
- Sterilize your collection bottles.
- Sterilize your baby's feeding bottles.
- Do not use lanolin as a lubricant since it will keep your nipples moist which can encourage yeast growth.[3]
- Consider necessary changes to your diet.

Blocked Ducts

A blockage in a milk duct can occur when lactating and many women who are exclusively pumping will experience blocked ducts. Some women will find they are highly prone to blocked ducts, and, if this is the case with you, take this into consideration when dropping pumps sessions or weaning. Symptoms of a blocked duct include soreness or pain in a localized area of your breast, redness around the area, a hard lump that can vary in size depending on how large the blockage is, and a decrease in milk volume.

It is extremely important to resolve a block as soon as possible since it can lead to mastitis if not dealt with. Try to avoid blocked ducts by removing as much milk as possible from your breasts as often as possible. Do not make sudden or drastic alterations to your pumping schedule, and do not wear tight, restrictive bras or underwire bras.

Treatment for blocked ducts includes the following:

- Pump! Pump often and longer if necessary to work out the blockage.
- Massage the affected area prior to and while pumping.
- Use breast compressions while pumping. Do not be overly forceful, however, since you can damage breast tissue.
- Use heat on the affected area. Take a hot shower before pumping or use a warm compress on the site.
- After pumping, you can use cold compresses to reduce the inflammation and discomfort.
- If there is a blister on the nipple, you may need to lance it with a sterile needle in order to free the blockage.

- In stubborn cases, ultrasound may work to break up the blockage. Speak to your doctor or a physiotherapy clinic.
- Lecithin capsules also benefit some women. These may be worth considering if you are prone to blocked ducts. It is believed that lecithin reduces the viscosity of breast milk.[4]
- Try castor oil compresses to reduce inflammation and remove the blockage. Use a small piece of clean cloth, folded over a few times. Soak the cloth with castor oil and warm it in a microwave. Be careful not to heat it to the point where it will burn your skin. Place the cloth over the blockage and then wrap the breast with plastic wrap. Finally, place a warm water bottle or heating pad over the breast. Allow this to sit in place for about twenty minutes and then remove. Wash your breast thoroughly to remove any remaining oil. You can keep the cloth in a plastic bag and reuse it. Repeat the compress two to three times a day until the blockage is cleared. One pumping mom shared with me that to make the use of castor oil even easier, she would soak a panty liner in castor oil and then adhere the sticky side to the inside of her bra. Apparently it worked like a charm!
- Another novel, anecdotal solution to stubborn blocked ducts is to use an electric toothbrush, facial brush, or hand-held massager to "massage" the area. The massage and vibrating action can help to release the block. No scientific data to back this one up, but it certainly can't hurt!

Mastitis

Mastitis is an infection of the breast. It can arise from a blocked duct if left untreated, but this is not always the cause. Symptoms are similar to a blocked duct but are usually more severe in terms of pain, inflammation, and redness. Mastitis is also often accompanied by a fever and overall sense of feeling unwell.

Treatment for mastitis includes the following:

- Mastitis will sometimes require a physician's intervention and treatment. Seek the advice of your doctor as soon as possible, especially if you have a high fever.
- Antibiotics are often required and will be prescribed by your doctor; however, some research suggests that using probiotics (in this particular study strains of Lactobacilli were used) instead of antibiotics can be an effective alternative with the study participants showing greater improvement and a reduced risk of reoccurrence of mastitis when compared to women who were treated with antibiotics.[5]
- Do not stop pumping since engorgement will worsen the symptoms and can result in blocked ducts, which will compound the situation even further.
- Check with your doctor to ensure the medication you are being prescribed is fully compatible with breastfeeding. Usually a suitable medication can be found.
- Rest as much as possible.
- Use heat on the area of infection prior to pumping, and cold compresses after pumping.

- Use ibuprofen for pain and inflammation or acetaminophen for pain.

Using a suction level on your pump that is too high

Using too high a suction level is one of the major causes of nipple trauma when pumping. Many women find that when they turn down the suction they actually increase their yield since it is more comfortable and often this will increase let-downs. Find the minimum suction level that will work for you. Some pumps will actually produce enough suction to seriously damage your breast! Don't assume that the pump is calibrated in such a way that the highest suction will work the best or even be safe.

Friction

Friction is a problem that can be easily avoided, but one that is not often mentioned to women who are pumping. The friction caused by a breast pump can definitely cause pain and soreness. The best line of defense is to use a lubricating product before you pump. Lanolin is one product that is often used (although remember that lanolin is contraindicated if you are suffering from a yeast infection). Olive oil and coconut oil are other recommended options and offer antibacterial, antiviral, and antifungal properties as well.[6, 7] Anecdotally, coconut oil works really well and this would likely be my go-to option if I were pumping today.

Another source of pain caused by friction can be flanges that are too small. If you have large nipples and find that they are squished into the flange tunnel or rubbing against the sides of the flanges when pumping, you may want to try a larger flange.

Conversely, flanges that are too big and that allow a large amount of the areola to be pulled into the flange when pumping can also cause pain and discomfort. If this is the case you can try a smaller flange, if available, or try a soft silicone insert that will reduce the diameter of the flange. To some extent, finding the right flange size is a bit of trial and error, so don't hesitate to try alternatives if what you're using is not working for you.

The Pump

As discussed in the chapter on breast pumps there is a wide variety of pumps on the market, all just a bit different in their operation. The suck and release cycles will vary by pump and manufacturer. If you have tried to remedy pain caused by pumping and have not found any success, consider trying a different pump.

There are other causes of pain during pumping such as Reynauld's syndrome, eczema, and other skin sensitivities. These, however, are best dealt with at your doctor's office.

In general, take good care of your breasts and nipples! Here are some general guidelines for breast care:

- Don't use soap on your breasts when bathing. It can be very drying and artificial fragrances may cause irritation.
- Change your breast pads regularly to avoid moisture sitting against your breasts for long periods. If using washable pads, be sure to dry them fully before using.
- Wash your clothes with a mild, fragrance-free detergent.
- Wash your bras regularly.
- Wear well-fitting, supportive bras to prevent unnecessary stretching of ligaments, and avoid underwire bras that can impinge on ducts.
- Leave some breast milk on your nipples after pumping and allow to air dry, which can assist in

warding off infections and help prevent dryness. Make use of the amazing properties of breast milk!

Lack of Sleep

Lack of sleep is certainly not unique to the life of a mom who is pumping exclusively; however, due to the extra time involved to pump and then bottle feed, there may seem to be fewer hours in a day. The time when your baby sleeps is a prime pumping opportunity, and in order to build a strong supply, it is important to pump during the night at least once (at least for the first few months), which means your night feeds become an hour or more in length—unless you can convince your partner to get up and feed the baby while you pump.

So how do you get sleep? Well, to some degree, you should probably resign yourself to the fact that you will be sleep deprived. I know, that's not what you wanted to hear, but there are a few other things you may consider:

- Enlist the help of anyone you can. If someone offers to take the baby while you pump, let them. If someone offers to cook dinner, let them. If someone offers to get you some groceries, let them. Is there a teenager in your neighbourhood who would enjoy spending some time with your baby, or even your older child, allowing you to get a bit of rest? Look at all possibilities.
- As we talked about in a previous chapter, talk to your family about what you are doing and what you need. Once people understand your situation a bit better they will be more inclined to offer help and limit the expectations they place on you.

- Sleep when you can and don't worry about the house. An amazing thing about a dirty house is that it will still be dirty when you wake up tomorrow and even next week. A clean house is not the sign of a good mother, but an exhausted mother. Take the time you need first, and don't give it to your house until all other important things are taken care of.

- Keep good sleep habits when possible. I know that sounds impossible, but try to keep some sort of regular bedtime schedule. Avoid eating late into the evening. Keep your bedroom conducive to sleep: draw the curtains, use soft light, and don't use the space to watch television or pay your bills.

- Let your partner take the night feeds occasionally or do the last evening feeding and put the baby to bed so that you can go to bed early. Even if you only do this once in a while, the extra hour or two of sleep will feel amazing. Getting in a good night's sleep every once in a while will keep you sane.

- Remember that all moms are facing sleep deprivation right along with you. You are not alone! It will get better, I promise.

"Are You Breastfeeding?"

Even though it would seem that how you feed your baby should not be a concern to anyone outside of your family, invariably, someone will ask you if you are breastfeeding and often women who exclusively pump are uneasy or unsure of how to answer. How you respond to this question is really is up to you. You have two equally appropriate options:

- Answer "yes". This is probably the easiest and quickest answer; however, it may lead to quizzical looks when you pull out a bottle to feed your baby. But it is true—you are "breastfeeding by bottle".
- Accept any opportunity to tell people about the option of exclusively pumping and the fact that it is a viable alternative to formula feeding.

Your decision on how to handle this question is often determined by who is asking the question. In general, though, it is a positive thing to explain how beneficial breast milk is to an infant and how you are providing breast milk for your child. The option of exclusively pumping is still not widely known in our society. When we share our experience with others, we give them an opportunity to learn about this alternative to formula feeding and as a result more women will learn about exclusively pumping, more support will be given to pumping moms, and more babies will get their mothers' milk.

Challenges Continuing On

Yes, it is true, you may, at some point in time, resent your pump. You will look at it as though it is a living, breathing creature that has pushed its way into your life to destroy every spare moment you once had. You will often feel attached to your pump—physically attached to it, that is. You may even go so far as to cover it up with a large blanket so you don't have to look at it. This, I'm afraid, is all part of exclusively pumping.

When pregnant, I imagined what it would be like to leave the hospital with my newborn and take him home. However, when he was born at thirty-one weeks gestation things did not work out as planned. When I was released from the hospital three days after his birth, he did not come with me. Instead of leaving with my baby, I left with a breast pump. And the breast pump stayed with me for the next year. We (the pump and I, that is) had a kind of love-hate relationship—at least I'd like to think the pump had some feelings for me. There were times when I hated the sight of it and I remember the resignation I felt knowing that I needed to "hook up" to it instead of being able to go to bed. But I also loved the fact that it enabled me to nourish my son for the first year of his life.

The best advice I can give when you are feeling tied to your pump is to take it one pump at a time. Don't think about the long term, but think only of the present. Consider what this "contraption" is allowing you to do and what it is providing for your child. Take baby steps. Don't look at big goals, but instead set small, achievable goals. You may want to pump for a year, but if all you can do is pump for today and then reassess it tomorrow, that's okay. In the end, you will likely find that you continue much longer than you ever thought possible.

Another suggestion that might help you overcome feelings of resentment or discouragement is to become portable. Using a personal pump such as the Medela Pump In Style or Ameda Purely Yours can allow you to pump on the go. This kind of pump allows you to express milk pretty much anywhere—even when in the car. Also, using a nursing cover when pumping outside of the home can offer an additional level of privacy.

When you're having a rough day, just remember it does get easier. Early on, a frequent pumping schedule can make leaving the house seem like a monumental task and leave you with very little energy for anything else. By the time you pump, pack up, get your baby ready and yourself ready, it is almost time to pump again and leaving the house may hardly seem worth it—but this won't last for long. As you start dropping sessions, you will gain more time away from your pump, and you will gain the freedom you desire.

Caring for Your Baby While Pumping

Early on in your newborn's life, pumping will not be as difficult to fit in as it will be in a couple months' time. Although you have to pump often, hopefully your baby will be sleeping most of the day away with only brief alert periods and you will be able to pump while your baby is sleeping. Unfortunately, this makes it impossible to follow that ever present advice to sleep while your baby is sleeping, so be sure to care for yourself as much as possible and prioritize rest as much as you can, as we've discussed.

Once your baby gets three or four months under his or her belt, pumping will be a little easier since you will now be able to entertain your child with various devices and contraptions such as a bouncy chair, a baby video, an exersaucer, or a swing. Pumping that cannot be done during nap time can often be done while your baby entertains himself with one of these activities.

It is the months in between the newborn stage and the stage when your baby can entertain himself and enjoy investigating the world for awhile on his own—within a confined space of course—that will pose the greatest challenge to your pumping schedule. From about two months to four or five months, your baby will be awake for longer periods, perhaps be more resistant to napping, and look forward to more interaction from you to fill in the awake time. This can be stressful and exasperating when you need to pump but your baby's schedule will not work with yours.

First, know that this period will pass and, in most cases, you will soon have a child who is able to keep themselves entertained for short periods without too much trouble. You will also be able to drop sessions soon, which will allow you to stretch out the time between pumping sessions if needed. As well, it is important to understand that the number of pumping sessions in a day is probably more important than the length of time between sessions. If you are trying to fit six sessions into a day, don't worry about spacing them all exactly four hours apart. If, for example, you have pumped two hours ago and your baby falls asleep in the car on the way home and continues sleeping when you bring her in, then use this unexpected nap time to pump! Chances are you will have more difficulty doing it later once your little one wakes up. You will most likely find that the pumping session after only two hours has a slightly reduced yield, but the next pump (which will likely be after three or four hours) will produce a greater volume. In the end, all will usually even out. And remember that volumes should always be considered on the basis of a twenty-four hour period, not a single session.

Of course, another thing you must do is to accept help when it is offered. (Yes, I know this is a repeated refrain, but it is something that many moms are not good at.) It can be difficult enough just taking care of a new baby, but adding in pumping can make it overwhelming. Take people up on their offers to help out. As is discussed in the chapter about relationships, it is important to have an honest discussion with your spouse and share with him the importance to you of providing breast milk for your baby—he will probably share in your desire to feed your baby breast milk. Share your emotions and your needs with him so he can understand what you are going through. Share with him the ways in which he can support you in your decision to exclusively pump. The time you are pumping is a great opportunity for dad to get some one-on-one time with his new baby!

Most of all, recognize that you are not going to do this alone. Even if the help you receive is simply moral and emotional support, it will make a world of difference. A shoulder to cry on and a strong arm to pull you back up when you feel you can't continue will make a world of difference in trying to exclusively pump for the long haul. You are definitely not alone in this, so reach out and find some people who understand and who can cheer you on!

The Desire to Quit

If you never have this overwhelming desire to quit exclusively pumping, then I would suggest you're not human! Exclusively pumping is taxing—both mentally and physically. You are doing double duty when it comes to feeding your baby. Fortunately, the good days usually outnumber the bad days.

When one of the not-so-good days strike, first consider the reasons you are pumping. Often, simply remembering that you are doing this for the health of your child will be enough to get you through. For some women, the financial cost of switching to formula will also play into why they are choosing to pump. Sometimes it will simply be personal accomplishment that will keep you pumping. Another reason I believe some women persevere with exclusively pumping is as a means of working through a difficult breastfeeding experience—we'll talk more about this in the chapter on weaning.

One of the most important elements of successful pumping is building and using a support system. This may come from the internet, friends or family, a doctor or lactation consultant, or any other person to whom you can go for support. Ideally, this person will have some experience with exclusively pumping or breastfeeding and have knowledge about pumping. Use your support system. It is one of the biggest predictors of success with exclusively pumping. The desire to quit is often frustration with a particular situation instead of a genuine desire to wean.

Every woman will get to a point, though, when the thought of weaning starts entering her mind. It is at this point when you have to carefully survey the situation. Consider the following questions:

- Is the reason for considering weaning because of a certain situation or event in your life which will change or pass? If there is something specific causing you to consider weaning, perhaps you could, or should, wait until it passes in order to make a clear-headed decision. Try not to make a rash decision about weaning without considering the whole picture.

- How close are you to your long-term goal? Perhaps you have already passed your long-term goal. Perhaps you are close enough to it that, through a long weaning process, you will still meet it. Perhaps you will realize that your goal needs to be adjusted or that it is not as important as you once thought it was. Or perhaps you will recognize that you really want to achieve your goal.

- How will you feel if you decide to wean now? A certain amount of emotion over weaning is to be expected, but it should not consume you. Will you feel proud of yourself for pumping as long as you did? Or will you feel like you failed and didn't try hard enough? If possible, try to keep pumping long enough to work through these emotions before making a final decision.

- How much breast milk do you have in your freezer? Women with extremely large stashes in their freezer can feed breast milk for two months or more after they wean. This can allow you to wean a couple months ahead of your goal if you so desire and still meet your goal.

- How much support do you have to continue? Without a strong support system, it can be difficult to handle the daily pressures of pumping in addition to the pressures of life in general. You will need to look inside yourself and determine if you are able to continue on your own and if the benefits are worth the stress and other difficulties that you are facing. Weigh it carefully. Your child benefits from your milk, but he also benefits from a healthy and happy mommy.

- Do you feel as though you could continue if you had to? Often, we feel as though we simply cannot continue on, but this is rarely the case. Ask yourself the tough questions. Draw on your reserves. If you do not have any reserves on which to draw, then perhaps it is time to wean.

- Are you currently able to meet your baby's daily intake requirements? If you are not meeting your baby's daily intake, you may get to a point where you ask yourself if it is worth it. As always, only you can answer this. Any amount of breast milk provides significant value for your baby. However, if you are fighting to maintain your supply and feel you are losing the battle, you should allow yourself to consider how much more you would be able to give your baby if you were not pumping. Does it balance out or would not pumping provide more?

Indulging in a Glass or Two

Many moms who pump worry about drinking alcohol and question whether they need to "pump and dump" after they have consumed a drink or two. Although the American Academy of Pediatrics states that alcohol consumption should be limited to occasional intake and should not exceed 0.5 grams of alcohol per kilogram of body weight,[8] other experts such as Dr. Thomas Hale suggest that "mothers who ingest alcohol in moderate amounts can generally return to breastfeeding as soon as they feel neurologically normal."[9] As with most things, moderation is key. An occasional drink should not cause you to worry or require you to pump and dump. Alcohol will transfer through your breast milk, but less than 2% of the alcohol you drink will reach your milk.[10] It's best to avoid alcohol for the first couple months of your baby's life as a newborn's liver function is still immature and will have to work very hard to detoxify the alcohol.

Working and Exclusively Pumping

In our modern world, it is a simple fact that many new mothers need to return to work within their baby's first year, and often within the first few weeks or months. In some ways, the transition from exclusively pumping at home to exclusively pumping at work should not be too much of a problem. Unlike breastfeeding moms who have to balance breastfeeding while at home with pumping at work, your daily routine will be similar whether you are at home or at work. There are, though, challenges that can come up such as finding time in the day to pump, creating a viable system for expressed breast milk use with a daycare provider, and managing milk storage at work.

It is important to know that in many countries your rights as a breastfeeding mother are protected, and, in most cases, this means that you must be given time to pump during your workday. Open communication is always a good idea, so talk to your employer about your needs: time to pump, private location, fridge, sink. Know your rights, and although you can be considerate of your employer's needs, stand up for what *you* need, especially when you are backed by the support of your country's legislation.

Milk storage at work really is no different than milk storage at home. It is a good idea to label your milk and keep it separate from other food items in a shared kitchen; just to be sure someone doesn't grab your milk for their coffee! Depending on the length of your work day, you might be able to simply keep the milk in a cooler with a cold pack.

You should have access to a sink, but if washing up your pump flanges is challenging, you might choose to simply keep them in the fridge between pumping sessions or use cleansing wipes such as the Medela Quick Clean wipes.

If you find your milk supply is dropping during the work week due to a reduced pumping schedule, one solution to consider is power pumping over the weekends. This will help boost your supply a bit through the week.

Be sure to have a talk with your daycare provider and share the proper methods for using and storing expressed breast milk. It is important to label your milk with your baby's name, amounts, and date. You might consider using a wax pencil or labels. Labels, however, don't always clean off well.

This certainly isn't an exhaustive discussion of the challenges of working and pumping. Most information you'll find available centres around breastfeeding and pumping at work, and some of this information might be helpful even if you are exclusively pumping. There are numerous discussion boards for moms who are working and pumping. The book *Milk Memos*, published in 2007, is a fun and realistic look at pumping at work. Another book called *Working Without Weaning* provides practical advice for pumping at work, although with a focus on breastfeeding mothers.[11]

Chapter 13

An End and a New Beginning: Weaning

Weaning is quite simply the process of moving a baby to food other than its mother's milk. So for baby, weaning is a natural process which starts—albeit slowly—when she begins to eat solid foods; however, for mothers, this process also means slowing and eventually stopping lactation. For exclusively pumping moms, the weaning process must be controlled by the mother, in contrast to a breastfeeding mother who, if she chooses to let the baby self-wean, will have the baby control the process. And while weaning is largely about gradually stopping milk production, to some extent, weaning is about making peace with the past and moving on to a new future. Weaning can be an emotional period and it can be a freeing period; often it is both. Planning your weaning process, taking the time to contemplate your experience exclusively pumping, and reflecting on the reasons for exclusively pumping can help to make the experience of weaning pain-free and positive. In this chapter we'll talk about when to wean, the emotions that can arise, how to transition your baby off of breast milk, and the process of weaning.

When to Wean

When to wean is entirely up to you. Your breast milk will continue to provide important nutrients and calories for as long as you choose to feed it. While some women are able to drop down to only two pumps a day and produce enough breast milk to meet the needs of their babies, these women are decidedly not the majority.

Your decision to wean will likely take into account a number of elements: your long-term goal, your baby's health, your health, your family, your emotions, your work requirements, and a number of other individual factors. In many cases, the decision to wean is a gradual one. You will perhaps feel that it is time and will take a few weeks to test the waters and try to gauge just how you feel about the idea of no longer feeding your baby your milk.

Do take the time to make the decision. Once you start the process of weaning, it is difficult (but not impossible) to reverse it. Make the decision based on your needs but also based on your emotions. Many mothers feel they need to wean due to their personal situation, but emotionally they are unwilling to give it up. Do not discount your emotions, making a purely intellectual decision.

Consider why you want to wean. If you are feeling overwhelmed, perhaps simply dropping a pumping session will make enough of a difference and you will decide to continue pumping. If your supply is the issue, get advice on how to increase it. Read the suggestions in the previous chapter "The Ups and Downs of Pumping". Be informed. Ensure you are confident that you have tried everything you are willing to try. Whatever your reasons for weaning, be comfortable with your decision. Most women will feel at peace with their decision when the time is right.

It's a good idea to take your time when making decisions about weaning. I'd suggest setting a date for some time in the future to start the process. This will allow you time to sit with the decision and also give you the opportunity to change the date or the entire plan if you should decide that now is not the time to wean.

Guilt Associated With Weaning

Many women report feelings of guilt when they consider weaning. However, most women are able to move beyond these feelings and settle into an understanding that the time is right, recognizing that their feelings of guilt are more closely related to a sadness that they will no longer be providing breast milk for their baby. Think back to the chapter on guilt. Just as we sometimes label our feelings as guilt when we are unable to breastfeed, we may also label our emotions surrounding weaning as guilt; however, in both cases they may be more accurately labeled as grief.

You are coming to the end of a very important chapter in your relationship with your baby. Just as breastfeeding moms will feel a sense of loss when they wean their breastfed babies, I think it is just as normal for a pumping mom to feel loss. For the first months of your baby's life you were the sole or primary source of your baby's nutrition. Your body nourished your baby *in utero* and has continued to feed your baby after your baby's birth. Now he is growing older and weaning acknowledges this growth. Acknowledge your emotions, investigate them, work through any lingering sense of grief or loss you may feel if you had wanted to breastfeed, and then move on content with the job you've done and the love you've shown to your baby. Look how big, strong, and healthy your baby has grown—you've done that!

This is one of the rites of motherhood, and regardless of whether you are exclusively pumping or breastfeeding, or whether you wean at two months or two years, the emotions will be there. You will continue to feed your darling baby—both with food and with love—and be an incredible force in his life. Our roles merely change. They do not end—ever. After ten years of being connected to the community of exclusively pumping women, I can say that many women relate to pumping as a way to control an uncontrollable situation and a way to work through the loss of the breastfeeding relationship that so many of us wanted. When we wean, it may feel as though that control is now lost to us. But you are simply moving into a new experience of parenting. Take some time to remember the incredible things you have done over the past few months! Deal with the sad and painful, too. And then move forward proudly, ready to accept the next challenges of motherhood.

Not Yet Ready to Wean?

Perhaps you are not yet ready to wean. Possibly you are weaning because of pressure to do so from friends or family members. Maybe you are weaning because you are returning to work and do not feel you can continue to pump when working. Perhaps you need to start a medication and have been told it is contraindicated while breastfeeding. In all these cases, perhaps you should continue to pump.

If you are simply not prepared to stop pumping and want to continue feeding your baby breast milk, then do so. Drop a session, alter your work load, or enlist the help of friends and family. Do whatever it takes to continue until *you* feel it is the right time to wean.

If your family or friends are pressuring you to wean, ignore them. Do what you want to do. It is your body and your baby. You are doing what you know is best for your child and you will also wean when you know it is best for you and your child.

If you are returning to work, there is no reason you need to wean. Employers are becoming more and more supportive of breastfeeding mothers and many large companies are even establishing pumping rooms and supplying fridges to store expressed breast milk. Speak to your employer about your needs to see if you can work out an arrangement. Most countries now recognize the rights of breastfeeding mothers and require employers to provide breaks for pumping and appropriate facilities (read: not the bathroom). While it may require a little more effort and planning on your part, it is possible to work and pump.

If you need to start a new medication and are concerned about the possible effects on your baby, seek expert advice. Visit www.motherisk.org or www.infantrisk.com. While some medications are clearly not compatible with breastfeeding, some have minimal risks to the baby and, through careful consultation with your doctor and your child's doctor, you may decide it is beneficial for your baby to continue to receive breast milk and that the risk is acceptable. Or you may be able to find an alternative drug therapy that will not affect your breast milk. Do not wean until you are entirely satisfied that you have learned about all your options.

Making the Switch

When you decide that it's time to wean, it is important to consider how you'll switch from breast milk to an alternative source of nutrition before you begin your weaning process (or at least before your freezer stash runs out if you are fortunate enough to have one). Speak with your baby's doctor about the best replacement for breast milk. Depending on your baby's age and requirements, you may need to consider specialty formulas or you may be able to switch to whole cow's milk if your baby is old enough and eating a wide variety of solids. You may even choose to skip cow's milk altogether. Your child's doctor will be able to provide advice specific to your baby's needs.

Many women are concerned that their babies may not accept the new food, whether it is formula or cow's milk. If you plan on switching to formula, you may feel more comfortable starting the weaning process if you know your baby will accept formula. Offer a bottle or two and see what happens. Many babies don't even notice there is something different in the bottle, and if this is the case for your child, it can make you more comfortable with the idea of weaning. When switching over to formula, do it gradually. Ask your child's doctor for her recommendation on how best to do it.

If your baby is not accepting of formula, you may consider slowly introducing the formula by mixing it with expressed breast milk. This slow introduction should also be done with whole cow's milk. Offer your baby's regular bottles mixed with 30 milliliters (1 ounce) of formula or cow's milk. Wait a day or two and then add another 30 milliliters (1 ounce) while reducing the amount of breast milk. Watch your baby for any signs that the cow's milk or formula is not being tolerated well. Continue to add more formula or cow's milk and reduce the amount of expressed breast milk. Within a week or two, the substitution should be complete.

How to Wean

The process of weaning is actually quite simple and relates directly to how your supply is established and maintained. What you will be doing is everything you have avoided while you have been pumping, and you will be starting to do the things you were warned not to do. It's not often in life that you get to break all the rules!

Allow yourself enough time to do a slow, gradual wean. Do not expect to be finished on a set date. Instead, allow your body to dictate the schedule. The more slowly you wean, the fewer negative effects you will have from it. By slowly weaning, you can have a comfortable and easy end to your pumping experience.

Most women will only be pumping three or four times a day when they decide to wean. If you are pumping more, it will take longer for you to go through the process. Review, if necessary, how milk is produced and what processes are in place that maintain or increase supply. During weaning, you will be leaving milk in your breasts instead of removing as much as you usually would. This will signal your body to slow down and eventually stop production. You will also start to lengthen the time between pumping sessions.

The Process

- The first step is to begin reducing the length of time you are pumping each session. Do not dramatically cut your sessions; instead, start by reducing the time you pump by three to five minutes at the most. See how your body responds.
- After a couple of days, continue to reduce the length of your pumping sessions. Once again, only decrease the time by a few minutes. Don't make big changes at this point.
- You should start to see a small decline in your supply simply by reducing the length of time you are pumping.
- Continue to slowly reduce the length of sessions; ensure no hard spots or blocked ducts develop. If they do, it is important to work them out with massage and compressions, warm compresses prior to pumping, and perhaps the use of a castor oil compress.

- Your next step is to begin stretching the amount of time between your pumping sessions as you would if you wanted to drop a pumping session. However, your goal is to eventually eliminate all sessions, so it is best not to get overly concerned about your pumping schedule by trying to pump at specific times. Instead, let your body start to guide you as to when you need to pump. Do not pump immediately when you start to feel full; instead wait for another hour or so. It's important not to allow yourself to become overly engorged, but do stretch out the time within comfortable limits.

- As you continue to reduce the length of your pumping sessions, your supply should start decreasing and you will be able to comfortably go longer between pumps.

- Switch from a scheduled pumping regime to only pumping when you feel you need to. When you start to feel pressure or get engorged, pump. If you feel any hard spots developing, pump.

- If you are prone to blocked ducts or mastitis, take the weaning process very slowly! Pump to relieve the pressure as soon as it starts to develop, but do not pump to "empty" unless this is the only way to remove a block.

- The key at this stage is to pump only to relieve any fullness in your breasts or to release any hard spots. You must leave milk in your breasts. This is the only way to wean.

- Depending on how many pumping sessions you were doing when you started to wean, you will most likely see a dramatic decrease in your supply when you drop to around two sessions a day. Every woman is different though, so do not worry if your weaning experience is different than someone else's. Simply ensure that you are reducing the amount of time you are pumping and lengthening the time between pumping sessions. Stay focused on your weaning plan and don't be in a hurry to finish.

- Eventually you will get to a point where you only need to pump once a day and then you will be able to go thirty-six hours and then forty-eight hours and then you will perhaps be able to go five or even seven days before needing to pump again.

- Most women, once they have arrived at this point, find that they do need to pump at least once after a week or so. If you are having any tenderness or pressure in your breasts, it is best to pump for a very short time—five or ten minutes—just to relieve the discomfort. This is usually the last time you will need to pump.

- Your breasts will continue to produce small amounts of milk for several weeks, or even months, and if you try, you may be able to hand express small drops. Eventually, this too will end.

If you start to wean from two or three pumping sessions a day, you can expect the process to take approximately two to three weeks. If you are starting the weaning process with a extremely large supply or a frequent pumping schedule, be prepared for it to take you a bit longer. It's best to be patient and not to rush it. It will happen; believe in the process.

Relief for Engorgement and Discomfort

It should be your goal during the weaning process to avoid engorgement and discomfort; however, it may be impossible in some cases. If you do experience soreness or engorgement, try the following suggestions to relieve your discomfort:

- Use cold compresses to relieve the swelling.
- Use a pain reliever such as acetaminophen or ibuprofen.
- Wear a supportive, well-fitting bra but do not wear one with an underwire and do not bind your breasts since this can encourage blocked ducts to develop.
- Try putting chilled, green cabbage leaves in your bra for approximately 20 minutes several times a day.
- Consider using herbs such as dried sage, jasmine, peppermint, spearmint, lemon balm, or oregano to reduce your milk supply.[1]
- You may have avoided the use of hormonal birth control while pumping, but it is okay to start using it now. It may cause a reduction in your supply. However, I certainly wouldn't start taking hormonal birth control for this purpose alone.
- The decongestant pseudoephedrine, found in numerous over-the-counter cold and allergy medications, can, as one of its side effects, reduce milk supply. It is passed through breast milk though so you may need to pump and dump any milk you express while taking it. Check with your pharmacist.
- Most importantly, go slowly! You should have very little, if any, discomfort when weaning.

The After-Effects of Weaning

Once you have weaned, give yourself time to adjust to your new life. It can feel very strange to no longer have your time strictly scheduled. Enjoy your regained freedom and take some time to reflect on your accomplishments.

Once you have weaned, your period should return if it has not already. It may take a few months for your cycle to normalize. And you may find that you have heavier periods than before you were pregnant. This is completely normal.

After weaning, your breasts may actually be smaller than their pre-pregnancy size. This is also normal since the milk-producing glands replaced the fatty tissue in the breasts during lactation and now those glands are involuting.

You may also find that your emotions are much more on edge as your hormone levels return to their non-lactating, non-pregnancy state. During lactation, your estrogen levels are very low and once you wean they should return to their pre-pregnancy state.

Your appetite may also change. Often it will decrease. You may need to be more careful about what you are eating since it will be much easier to gain weight now that you are no longer expending the extra energy required to produce milk.

In general, give yourself time to relax and reflect on your experience exclusively pumping. No doubt you have seen in your baby the benefits of your decision, and you will continue to see them for years to come. It is an experience that rarely leaves a woman unchanged. You have most likely grown and recognized your strength and your ability to do what you feel is best for you and your family. Enjoy your baby; they don't stay babies for long.

Chapter 14

An Invitation

The most common statement I hear from women who are exclusively pumping is "I didn't know this was a 'thing'!" or another variation, "I thought I was the only one doing it!" While the knowledge and acceptance of exclusively pumping have definitely increased over the past several years, it is still largely an unknown option. Together we can work to ensure other women know that exclusively pumping is an option for them and, if they choose this path, that they are not alone.

Although it is often argued that women are choosing to exclusively pump instead of breastfeed, this is not in line with what I've experienced. I would argue that most women who exclusively pump desperately wanted to breastfeed but for one reason or another were unable to. The reality is that women are choosing to exclusively pump instead of feed formula. Ideally, all new mothers and babies would receive meaningful breastfeeding education and support; our society would embrace breastfeeding mothers and work to remove barriers that make breastfeeding difficult; and we would learn about breastfeeding from observing our mothers, aunts, sisters, and friends, creating a breastfeeding culture that is merely a normal part of our larger culture. Unfortunately, we are not there yet. But while we wait for society to reach that point, in the meantime, I would invite you to join me in supporting, encouraging, and advocating for other women.

My first invitation is for you to join me on my website and the book's Facebook page: www.exclusivelypumping.com and www.facebook.com/exclusivelypumping. Reach out and connect with me and other women there. My goal is always to keep the page and message encouraging and supportive, a place without judgment, and a place that recognizes the simple fact that we are all doing the best we can for our children. Please consider joining us there.

My second invitation is for you to share your experience with those you meet who have the power to change the perception of exclusively pumping and who have the ability to encourage and support other women who may benefit from the knowledge that there is an alternative to formula when breastfeeding doesn't work out. Talk to your doctor, your baby's pediatrician, your lactation consultant. Sadly, many women are still being told that exclusively pumping isn't possible and that they will never maintain their milk supply if they choose this route. How many babies lose out on their mothers' milk as a result of this poor support and information? We know this isn't the reality of exclusively pumping, but we need to share this with those who have the opportunity to in turn share it with new moms. Identify yourself—as a proud exclusively pumping mom—to anyone who will listen and know that by doing so you'll be increasing awareness of exclusively pumping as an alternative to formula and helping other mothers access better information and support.

My final invitation is for you to share your experience with other moms. Exclusively pumping can be isolating on both a physical and social level. Not only are many women physically isolated in their home, but the lack of knowledge and acceptance of exclusively pumping creates a social isolation. If you are the only pumping mom in a room full of mothers it is easy to feel the odd "man" out. But there are others who are pumping; you just have to find them. Speak up, share your experience, and you may be surprised to find other women who are, like you, exclusively pumping to provide breast milk for their babies. Not only might you find camaraderie, but you may also provide support to another mother who also needs understanding— understanding that only another exclusively pumping mom can offer.

Whatever circumstances led you to exclusively pump for your baby, and regardless of how long you pump, I want you to know that you are a rock star! This option isn't for the faint of heart and yet I haven't met a single woman who regrets exclusively pumping for her baby. Your journey won't be without challenges, but as with all valuable pursuits, the rewards are immense. Remember to care for yourself through it all. Remember to honour the emotions you feel as a result of breastfeeding challenges and the loss of expectations about breastfeeding. But most of all, remember the strength and determination you have shown. You are a great mother!

Acknowledgements

No book project is completed by just one person, and this project has had many hands involved. I am grateful to the many women I've had the pleasure to communicate with over the past ten years and who have continued to support my efforts, my writing, and my websites. Some have become close friends, and it is these women who continue to motivate and inspire me.

A special thank you to Erin. While she likely doesn't realize it, her support early on was especially meaningful. Her passion and dedication to her children are fierce, and, as another mother runner, her strength and motivation amaze me.

Thank you to Christina and Kathy for reading an early version of this edition and providing honest, knowledgeable feedback. Your time and thoughtfulness mean a great deal to me.

A big thank you to Diane. Again another wonderful cover that perfectly captures the love and care all exclusively pumping mothers feel and express for their babies on a daily basis. I appreciate your expert guidance.

And as always, thank you to my family, especially my children, Graeme and Elizabeth, who continually amaze me. You're the reason I share my story with the world, and you are the reason I continue working to make breastfeeding a normal and accepted method of nurturing and nourishing infants in our society.

Endnotes and References

Chapter 1—The Alternative to Formula

1. *Global Strategy on Infant and Young Child Feeding,* World Health Organization, 2003. http://whqlibdoc.who.int/publications/2003/9241562218.pdf
2. ibid.
3. One way to find a lactation consultant near you is to use the "Find a Lactation Consultant" search feature on the International Lactation Consultant Association website: www.ilca.org.

Chapter 2—Making the Decision

1. *Global Strategy on Infant and Young Child Feeding,* World Health Organization, 2003. http://whqlibdoc.who.int/publications/2003/9241562218.pdf

Chapter 3—The Emotions of Exclusively Pumping

1. Diane Wiessinger, "Watch Your Language," *Journal of Human Lactation,* 12(1): 1-4 (1996).
2. For further discussion of lack of support, lack of information, and societal pressures and influence see *Breastfeeding, Take Two* by Stephanie Casemore.
3. Jessica Restaino, "Drained" in *Unbuttoned: Women Open Up About the Pleasures, Pains, and Politics of Breastfeeding,* 148.
4. Jessica Restaino, "Drained" in *Unbuttoned: Women Open Up About the Pleasures, Pains, and Politics of Breastfeeding,* 146.

Chapter 4—Lactation and Breast Milk Composition

1. The Academy of Medicine Protocol Committee, "ABM Clinical Protocol #9: Use of Galactogogues in Initiating or Augmenting the Rate of Maternal Milk Secretion," *Breastfeeding Medicine*, 6(1): 41-49 (2011).

2. Liliane Assairi, Claude Delouis, Pierre Gaye, Louis-Marie Houdebine, Michèle Ollivier-Bousquet, and Robert Denamur, "Inhibition by Progesterone of the Lactogenic Effect of Prolactin in the Pseudopregnant Rabbit," *Biochemical Journal*, 144(2): 245–252 (November 1974).

3. K. Uvnas-Moberg, "Oxytocin may mediate the benefits of positive social interaction and emotions," Psychoneuroendocrinology, 23 (8): 819-835 (November 1998).

4. Kelly Bonyata, "How does milk production work?" Kellymom, http://kellymom.com/pregnancy/bf-prep/milkproduction

5. Mark D. Cregan, Leon R. Mitoulas, Peter E. Hartmann, "Milk prolactin, feed volume and duration between feeds in women breastfeeding their full-term infants over a 24 h period," *Experimental Physiology*, 87 (2): 207-214 (March 2002).

6. Peter E. Hartmann, Robyn A. Owens, David B. Cox, *and* Jacqueline C. Kent, "Breast Development and Control of Milk Synthesis," *Food and Nutrition Bulletin*, Vol. 17, No. 4 (December 1996), http://archive.unu.edu/unupress/food/8F174e/8F174E02.htm

7. Steven E. J. Daly, Jacqueline C. Kent, Robyn A Owens, and Peter Hartmann, "Frequency and Degree of Milk Removal and the Short-term Control of Human Milk Synthesis," *Experimental Physiology*, 81: 861-875 (September 1996).

8. Jacqueline C. Kent, Leon R. Mitoulas, Mark D. Cregan, Donna T. Ramsay, Dorota A. Doherty, and Peter Hartmann, "Volume and Frequency of Breastfeedings and Fat Content of

Breast Milk Throughout the Day," *Pediatrics*, 117 (3):e387-e395 (March 2006).

9. ibid.

10. Steven E. J. Daly, Jacqueline C. Kent, Robyn A Owens, and Peter Hartmann, "Frequency and Degree of Milk Removal and the Short-term Control of Human Milk Synthesis," *Experimental Physiology*, 81: 861-875 (September 1996).

11. Kelly Bonyata, "How does milk production work?" Kellymom, http://www.kellymom.com/bf/supply/milk

12. Jacqueline C. Kent, Leon Mitoulas, David B. Cox, Robyn A. Owens, and Peter Hartmann, "Breast Volume and Milk Production During Extended Lactation in Women," *Experimental Physiology*, 84: 435-447 (March 1999).

13. ibid.

14. J. M. Morse, G. Ewing, D. Gamble , P. Donahue, "The effect of maternal fluid intake on breast milk supply: a pilot study," *Canadian Journal of Public Health Revue Canadienne de Sante Publique.* 83(3): 213-216 (May-June 1992).

15. Jacqueline C. Kent, Leon R. Mitoulas, Mark D. Cregan, Donna T. Ramsay, Dorota A. Doherty, and Peter Hartmann, "Volume and Frequency of Breastfeedings and Fat Content of Breast Milk Throughout the Day," *Pediatrics*, 117 (3):e387-e395 (March 2006).

16. ibid.

17. Katherine Isselmann DiSantis, Eric A. Hodges, and Jennifer Orlet Fisher, "The association of breastfeeding duration with later maternal feeding styles in infancy and toddlerhood: a cross-sectional analysis," *International Journal of Behavioral Nutrition and Physical Activity*, 10 (53) (April 2013).

18. R. Li, J. Magadia, S.B. Fein, L.M. Grummer-Strawn, "Risk of bottle-feeding for rapid weight gain during the first year of life," *Archives of Pediatric and Adolescent Medicine*, 166 (5): 431-436 (May 2012).

19. R.A. Crow, J.N. Fawcett, and P. Wright, "Maternal Behaviour During Breast- and Bottle-Feeding," *Journal of Behavioral Medicine*, 3 (3): 259-277 (September 1980).

20. Native Mothering, "An Explanation of The Enteromammary Secretory HostImmune System: How a Mother's Immune System is Shared Through Breast Milk," www.nativemothering.com/2010/08/an-explanation-of-the-enteromammary-secretory-host-immune-system/

21. "Pregnancy, Lactation, and Bone Health," National Institute of Arthritis and Musculoskeletal and Skin Disorders, www.niams.nih.gov/Health_Info/Bone/Bone_Health/Pregnancy/default.asp

Chapter 5—Exclusively Pumping 101: The Basics

1. D.K. Prime, C.P. Garbin, P.E. Hartmann, J.C. Keng, "Simultaneous breast expression in breastfeeding women is more efficacious than sequential breast expression," *Breastfeeding Medicine*, 7(6):442-447 (December 2012).

2. An excellent video showing hand expression technique: http://newborns.stanford.edu/Breastfeeding/HandExpression.html.

3. "Mix of Hand Techniques, Electric Pumping May Increase Milk Production in Mothers of Preterm Infants,"*Medscape*, July 23, 2009.

4. Two such products are Blossumz Soothing Breast Therapy Packs and the Nuk Breast Therapy Warm or Cool Relief Pack.

5. For a good source of information on baby carriers go to www.thebabywearer.com

6. "Caprylic Acid in Coconut Oil," *Livestrong.com*, October 1, 2010.

7. Michel Odent, "The Role of the Shy Hormone in Breastfeeding," published on Lactnet August 22, 2011.

8. Michel Odent, "The Role of the Shy Hormone in Breastfeeding," published on Lactnet August 22, 2011.

9. D.K. Prime, D.T. Geddes, A.R. Hepworth, N.J. Trengove, P.E. Hartmann, "Comparison of the patterns of milk ejection during repeated breast expression sessions in women," *Breastfeeding Medicine*, 6: 183-190 (August 2011).

10. http://www.d-mer.org/Mechanism_of_D-MER.html

11. ibid.

12. Jacqueline C. Kent, Leon R. Mitoulas, Mark D. Cregan, Donna T. Ramsay, Dorota A. Doherty, and Peter Hartmann, "Volume and Frequency of Breastfeedings and Fat Content of Breast Milk Throughout the Day," *Pediatrics*, 117 (3):e387-e395 (March 2006).

13. Jacqueline C. Kent, Leon Mitoulas, David B. Cox, Robyn A. Owens, and Peter Hartmann, "Breast Volume and Milk Production During Extended Lactation in Women," *Experimental Physiology*, 84: 435-447 (March 1999).

14. Steven E. J. Daly, Jacqueline C. Kent, Robyn A. Owens, and Peter Hartmann, "Frequency and Degree of Milk Removal and the Short-term Control of Human Milk Synthesis," *Experimental Physiology*, 81: 861-875 (September 1996).

15. J. Morton, R.J. Wong, J.Y. Hall, W.W. Pang, C.T. Lai, J. Lui, P.E. Hartmann, W.D. Rhine, "Combining Hand Techniques with Electric Pumping Increases the Caloric Content of Milk in Mothers of Preterm Infants," *Journal of Perinatology*, 32(10): 791-796 (October 2012).

16. J. Morton, J.Y. Hall, R.J. Wong, L. Thairu, W.E. Benitz, W.D. Rhine, "Combining Hand Techniques with Electric Pumping Increases Milk Production in Mothers of Preterm Infants," *Journal of Perinatology*, 29(11): 757-764 (November 2009).

17. A. Hörnell, C. Aarts, E. Kylberg, Y. Hofvander, M. Gebre-Medhin, "Breastfeeding Patterns in Exclusively Breastfed

Infants: A Longitudinal Prospective Study in Uppsala, Sweden," *Acta Paediatrica*, 88(2): 203-11 (February 1999).

18. Jacqueline C. Kent, Leon Mitoulas, David B. Cox, Robyn A. Owens, and Peter Hartmann, "Breast Volume and Milk Production During Extended Lactation in Women," *Experimental Physiology*, 84: 435-447 (March 1999).

19. "Mix of Hand Techniques, Electric Pumping May Increase Milk Production in Mothers of Preterm Infants,"*Medscape*, July 23, 2009.

20. www.motherisk.org

Chapter 6—The Next Step: Pumping Long Term

1. As a first stop for support, visit this book's Facebook page at www.facebook.com/exclusivelypumping.

Chapter 7—The Ups and Downs of Pumping: Increasing and Decreasing Supply

1. Pilar Codoñer-Franch, Maria T. Hernández-Aguilar, Almudena Navarro-Ruiz, Ana B. López-Jaén, Cintia Borja-Herrero, and Victoria Valls-Bellés, "Diet Supplementation During Early Lactation With Non-Alcoholic Beer Increases the Antioxidant Properties of Breastmilk and Decreases the Oxidative Damage in Breastfeeding Mothers," *Breastfeeding Medicine*, 8 (2): 164-169 (April 2013).

2. The Academy of Medicine Protocol Committee, "ABM Clinical Protocol #9: Use of Galactogogues in Initiating or Augmenting the Rate of Maternal Milk Secretion," *Breastfeeding Medicine*, 6(1): 41-49 (2011).

3. ibid.

4. ibid.

5. www.kellymom.com

6. The Academy of Medicine Protocol Committee, "ABM Clinical Protocol #9: Use of Galactogogues in Initiating or

Augmenting the Rate of Maternal Milk Secretion," *Breastfeeding Medicine*, 6(1): 41-49 (2011).

7. ibid.

8. ibid.

9. Jack Newman, "Domperidone, Getting Started," International Breastfeeding Centre, 2009, www.nibc.ca.

10. The Academy of Medicine Protocol Committee, "ABM Clinical Protocol #9: Use of Galactogogues in Initiating or Augmenting the Rate of Maternal Milk Secretion," *Breastfeeding Medicine*, 6(1): 41-49 (2011).

11. "Reglan," Drugs.com

12. The Academy of Medicine Protocol Committee, "ABM Clinical Protocol #9: Use of Galactogogues in Initiating or Augmenting the Rate of Maternal Milk Secretion," *Breastfeeding Medicine*, 6(1): 41-49 (2011).

13. "Domperidone," Drugs.com

14. The Academy of Medicine Protocol Committee, "ABM Clinical Protocol #9: Use of Galactogogues in Initiating or Augmenting the Rate of Maternal Milk Secretion," *Breastfeeding Medicine*, 6(1): 41-49 (2011).

15. Thanks to Noel Trujillo for her permission to print her recipe for Housepoet's Famous Lactation Boosting Cookies.

16. For more information about milk banking in North America see the Human Milk Banking Association of North America's website: www.hmbana.org.

17. Eats on Feets website is at www.eatsonfeets.org, and Human Milk 4 Human Baby's website can be found at www.hm4hb.net.

18. "Why Use Donor Milk?" Human Milk Banking Association of North America, https://www.hmbana.org/faq#why.

19. Eats on Feets website is at www.eatsonfeets.org, and Human Milk 4 Human Baby's website can be found at www.hm4hb.net.

Chapter 8—Pumps and Kits, Oh My!

1. D.K. Prime, C.P. Garbin, P.E. Hartmann, J.C. Keng, "Simultaneous breast expression in breastfeeding women is more efficacious than sequential breast expression," *Breastfeeding Medicine*, 7(6):442-447 (December 2012).

2. "Understanding the International Code," The International Baby Food Action Network, http://www.ibfan.org/issue-international_code-understant.html.

3. Helen C. Armstrong and Ellen Sokel, "The International Code of Marketing of Breast Milk Substitutes: What It Means for Mothers and Babies Worldwide," International Lactation Consultants Association, 2001.

4. The International Baby Food Action Network (IBFAN), www.ibfan.org.

5. "On the Trail of Code Compliancy," Kellymom, http://kellymom.com/bf/advocacy/trail-of-code-compliancy/.

6. Michael J. Zinamen, John T. Queenan, Miriam H. Labbock, Barrie Albertson, Vergie Hughes, "Acute Prolactin and Oxytocin Responses and Milk Yield to Infant Suckling and Artificial Methods of Expression in Lactating Women," Pediatrics, 89 (3): 437-440 (March 1992).

7. E. Jones, P. Dimmock, and S. Spencer, "A Randomised Controlled Trial to Compare Methods of Milk Expression After Preterm Delivery," *Archives of Disease in Childhood Neonatal Edition*, 85(2): F91-F95 (September 2001).

8. J. Morton, R.J. Wong, J.Y. Hall, W.W. Pang, C.T. Lai, J. Lui, P.E. Hartmann, W.D. Rhine, "Combining Hand Techniques with Electric Pumping Increases the Caloric Content of Milk in Mothers of Preterm Infants," *Journal of Perinatology*, 32(10): 791-796 (October 2012).

9. An excellent video showing hand expression technique: http://newborns.stanford.edu/Breastfeeding/HandExpression.html.

10. "Medical Devices: Buying and Renting a Breast Pump," U.S. Food and Drug Administration, www.fda.gov.

11. Nancy Mohrbacher, "Are Used Breast Pumps a Good Option: Issues to Consider," *LEAVEN*, 40(3): 54-55 (June-July 2004).

12. Michael W. Woolridge, "The 'Anatomy' of Infant Sucking," Health e-Learning, www.health-e-learning.com.

13. J. Hopkinson, W. Heird, "Maternal Response to Two Electric Breast Pumps," *Breastfeeding Medicine*, 4(1): 17-23 (March 2009).

14. "On the Trail of Code Compliancy," Kellymom, http://kellymom.com/bf/advocacy/trail-of-code-compliancy/.

15. Human Milk Banking Association of North America, "Best Practice for Expressing, Storing and Handling Human Milk in Hospitals, Homes and Child Care Settings," (2005).

16. R.A. Lawrence, "Storage of Human Milk and the Influence of Procedures on Immunological Components of Human Milk," *Actra Paediatrica*, 88(S430): 14-18 (September 1999).

Chapter 9—Feeding Baby

1. R.A. Lawrence, "Storage of Human Milk and the Influence of Procedures on Immunological Components of Human Milk," *Actra Paediatrica*, 88(S430): 14-18 (September 1999).

2. Susan Orlando, "The Immunologic Significance of Breast Milk," *Journal of Obsetric, Gynecologic, and Neonatal Nursing*, 24(7): 678-683 (September 1995).

3. The Academy of Medicine Protocol Committee, "ABM Clinical Protocol #8: Human Milk Storage Information for Home Use for Full-Term Infants," *Breastfeeding Medicine*, 5(3): 127-130 (2010).

4. Susan Orlando, "The Immunologic Significance of Breast Milk," *Journal of Obsetric, Gynecologic, and Neonatal Nursing*, 24(7): 678-683 (September 1995).

5. ibid.

6. The Academy of Medicine Protocol Committee, "ABM Clinical Protocol #8: Human Milk Storage Information for Home Use for Full-Term Infants," *Breastfeeding Medicine*, 5(3): 127-130 (2010).

7. ibid.

8. Susan Orlando, "The Immunologic Significance of Breast Milk," *Journal of Obsetric, Gynecologic, and Neonatal Nursing*, 24(7): 678-683 (September 1995).

9. R.A. Lawrence, "Storage of Human Milk and the Influence of Procedures on Immunological Components of Human Milk," *Actra Paediatrica*, 88(S430): 14-18 (September 1999).

10. Susan Orlando, "The Immunologic Significance of Breast Milk," *Journal of Obsetric, Gynecologic, and Neonatal Nursing*, 24(7): 678-683 (September 1995).

11. R.A. Lawrence, "Storage of Human Milk and the Influence of Procedures on Immunological Components of Human Milk," *Actra Paediatrica*, 88(S430): 14-18 (September 1999).

12. Susan Orlando, "The Immunologic Significance of Breast Milk," *Journal of Obsetric, Gynecologic, and Neonatal Nursing*, 24(7): 678-683 (September 1995).

13. R.A. Lawrence, "Storage of Human Milk and the Influence of Procedures on Immunological Components of Human Milk," *Actra Paediatrica*, 88(S430): 14-18 (September 1999).

14. Susan Orlando, "The Immunologic Significance of Breast Milk," *Journal of Obsetric, Gynecologic, and Neonatal Nursing*, 24(7): 678-683 (September 1995).

15. The Academy of Medicine Protocol Committee, "ABM Clinical Protocol #8: Human Milk Storage Information for Home Use for Full-Term Infants," *Breastfeeding Medicine*, 5(3): 127-130 (2010).

16. ibid.

17. ibid.

18. David J. Rechtman, Martin L. Lee, and H. Berg, "Effect of Environmental Conditions on Unpasteurized Donor Human Milk," *Breastfeeding Medicine*, 1(1): 24-26 (Spring 2006).

19. The Academy of Medicine Protocol Committee, "ABM Clinical Protocol #8: Human Milk Storage Information for Home Use for Full-Term Infants," *Breastfeeding Medicine*, 5(3): 127-130 (2010).

20. Susan Orlando, "The Immunologic Significance of Breast Milk," *Journal of Obsetric, Gynecologic, and Neonatal Nursing*, 24(7): 678-683 (September 1995).

21. R.A. Crow, J.N. Fawcett, and P. Wright, "Maternal Behaviour During Breast- and Bottle-Feeding," *Journal of Behavioral Medicine*, 3 (3): 259-277 (September 1980).

22. Access the WHO growth charts here: *www.cdc.gov/growthcharts/who_charts.htm*

23. R.A. Crow, J.N. Fawcett, and P. Wright, "Maternal Behaviour During Breast- and Bottle-Feeding," *Journal of Behavioral Medicine*, 3 (3): 259-277 (September 1980).

24. R. Li, J. Magadia, S.B. Fein, L.M. Grummer-Strawn, "Risk of bottle-feeding for rapid weight gain during the first year of life," *Archives of Pediatric and Adolescent Medicine*, 166 (5): 431-436 (May 2012).

25. Jacqueline C. Kent, Leon R. Mitoulas, Mark D. Cregan, Donna T. Ramsay, Dorota A. Doherty, and Peter Hartmann, "Volume and Frequency of Breastfeedings and Fat Content of Breast Milk Throughout the Day," *Pediatrics*, 117 (3): e387-e395 (March 2006).

26. Dee Kassing, "Bottle-feeding as a Tool to Reinforce Breastfeeding," *The Journal of Human Lactation*, 18(1): 56-60 (February 2002).

27. R.A. Lawrence, "Storage of Human Milk and the Influence of Procedures on Immunological Components of Human Milk," *Actra Paediatrica*, 88(S430): 14-18 (September 1999).

269

28. The Academy of Medicine Protocol Committee, "ABM Clinical Protocol #8: Human Milk Storage Information for Home Use for Full-Term Infants," *Breastfeeding Medicine*, 5(3): 127-130 (2010).

29. Jessica Sypolt, (September 17, 2008), Re: Can Diet Changes Help With Lipase Issues [Online Discussion Group]. Retrieved from http://forums.llli.org/showthread.php?59783-Can-diet-changes-help-with-the-Lipase-issue

30. Richard Quan, Christine Yang, Steven Rubenstein, Norman J. Lewiston, David K. Stevenson, John A. Kerner, Jr., "The Effect of Nutritional Additives on Anti-Infective Factors in Human Milk," *Clinical Pediatrics*, 33(6): 325-328 (June 1994).

31. Lourdes Sánchez, Miguel Calvo, Jeremy H. Brock, "Biological Role of Lactoferrin," *Archives of Disease in Childhood*, 67(5): 657-661 (May 1992).

32. Jan Riordan, *Breastfeeding and Human Lactation*, Sudbury: Jones and Bartlett Learning, 2009.

33. Susan Orlando, "The Immunologic Significance of Breast Milk," *Journal of Obsetric, Gynecologic, and Neonatal Nursing*, 24(7): 678-683 (September 1995).

34. World Health Organization, "Safe Preparation, Storage, and Handling of Powdered Infant Formula: Guidelines," World Health Organization, 2007.

35. Health Canada, "Recommendations for the Preparation and Handling of Powdered Infant Formula (PIFP)," Health Canada, 2010, online.

Chapter 10—Pumping and the NICU

1. Paula P. Meier, Janet L. Engstrom, Aloka L. Patel, Briana J. Jegier, Nicholas E. Bruns, "Improving the Use of Human Milk During and After the NICU Stay,"*Clinical Perinatology*, 37(1): 217-245 (March 2010).

2. Laurie Tarkan, "For Parents on NICU, Trauma May Last," *The New York Times*, August 25, 2009.

3. Lydia Furman, Nori Minich, Maureen Hack, "Correlates of Lactation in Mothers of Very Low Birth Weight Infants," *Pediatrics*, 109(4): 357 (April 2002).

4. J. Morton, J.Y. Hall, R.J. Wong, L. Thairu, W.E. Benitz, W.D. Rhine, "Combining Hand Techniques with Electric Pumping Increases Milk Production in Mothers of Preterm Infants," *Journal of Perinatology*, 29(11): 757-764 (November 2009).

5. ibid.

6. Stanford School of Medicine video of hand expression: http//:newborns.stanford.edu/Breastfeeding/HandExpression.html

7. J. Morton, R.J. Wong, J.Y. Hall, W.W. Pang, C.T. Lai, J. Lui, P.E. Hartmann, W.D. Rhine, "Combining Hand Techniques with Electric Pumping Increases the Caloric Content of Milk in Mothers of Preterm Infants," *Journal of Perinatology*, 32(10): 791-796 (October 2012).

8. N.J. Bergman, L.L. Linley, S.R. Fawcus, "Randomized Controlled Trial of Maternal-Infant Skin-to-Skin Contact from Birth Versus Conventional Incubator for Physiological Stabilization in 1200g to 2199g Newborns," *Acta Paediatrica*, 93(6): 779-785 (January 2007).

9. For further information about Kangaroo Care see www.kangaroomothercare.com.

10. N.J. Bergman, L.L. Linley, S.R. Fawcus, "Randomized Controlled Trial of Maternal-Infant Skin-to-Skin Contact from Birth Versus Conventional Incubator for Physiological Stabilization in 1200g to 2199g Newborns," *Acta Paediatrica*, 93(6): 779-785 (January 2007).

11. www.biologicalnurturing.com

12. ibid.

13. Mari Douma, "Baby-led Latching: An 'intuitive' approach to learning how to breastfeed," *Ontario Breastfeeding Committee Newsletter*, 4(4): 2-3 (December 2005).

Chapter 11—Relationships (With a Little Help from Your Friends)

1. *Mama's Milk* by Michael Elsohn, *What Baby Needs* by William Sears, *My Mommy's Warmth* by Anna Turner.

Chapter 12—You Can Do It! Overcoming Challenges

1. The Academy of Medicine Protocol Committee, "ABM Clinical Protocol #8: Human Milk Storage Information for Home Use for Full-Term Infants," *Breastfeeding Medicine*, 5(3): 127-130 (2010).
2. D.O. Ogbolu, A.A. Oni, O.A. Daini, A.P. Oloko, "In Virto Antimicrobial Properties of Coconut Oil on Candida Species in Ibadan, Nigeria," *Journal of Medicinal Food*, 10(2): 384-387 (June 2007).
3. See Dr. Jack Newman's "Yeast Protocol" at www.nbci.ca.
4. Kelly Bonyata, "Lecithin Treatment for Recurrent Plugged Ducts," www.kellymom.com
5. R. Arroyo, V. Martin, A. Maldonado, E. Jiménez, L. Fernández, J.M. Rodriguez, "Treatment of Infectious Mastitis During Lactation: antibiotics versus oral administration of Lactobacilli isolated from breast milk," *Clinical Infectious Diseases*, 50(12): 1551-1558 (June 2010).
6. Marek Doyle, "Caprylic Acid in Coconut Oil," Livestrong.com, October 1, 2010.
7. V.M. Verallo-Rowell, K.M. Dillague, B.S. Syah-Tjundawan, "Novel Antibacterial and Emollient Effects of Coconut and Virgin Olive Oils in Adult Atopic Dermatitis," *Dermatitis*, 19)6): 308-315 (November-December 2008).

8. Kelly Bonyata, "Breastfeeding and Alcohol," www.kellymom.com.

9. quotes in Kelly Bonyata, "Breastfeeding and Alcohol," www.kellymom.com.

10. Kelly Bonyata, "Breastfeeding and Alcohol," www.kellymom.com.

11. Cate Colburn-Smith and Andrea Serrette, *Milk Memos: How Real Moms Learned to Mix Business with Babies—and How You Can, Too* (2007); Kirsten Berggren, *Working Without Weaning: A working mother's guide to breastfeeding* (2006).

Chapter 13—An End and a New Beginning: Weaning

1. Kelly Bonyata, "Too Much Milk: Sage and Other Herbs for Decreasing Milk Supply," www.kellymom.com.

Index

Also by Stephanie Casemore

𝓑𝓻𝓮𝓪𝓼𝓽𝓯𝓮𝓮𝓭𝓲𝓷𝓰, Take Two
Successful Breastfeeding the Second Time Around

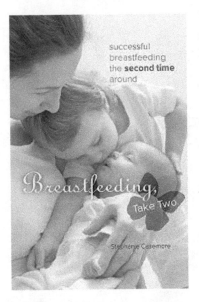

Breastfeeding is a biologically expected activity. It is, for many women, a relationship that is deeply desired, a relationship that is deeply emotional. To lose that relationship is to lose something very real, something that has value and purpose and meaning.

Breastfeeding Take Two: Successful Breastfeeding the Second Time Around examines the separation between biology and society and the balance that new mothers seek to find between the two. Written for women who have had previous breastfeeding challenges, *Breastfeeding, Take Two* will empower you to trust your body again, help you redefine what successful breastfeeding looks like, help you work through the emotions of your previous breastfeeding experience, provide information and advice to assist you in healing from the loss of your first breastfeeding experience, and position you for a successful experience—the second time around.

Visit the book's website at www.breastfeedingtaketwo.com and the Facebook page at www.facebook.com/breastfeedingtaketwo.

Now available in print and ebook formats.

CPSIA information can be obtained
at www.ICGtesting.com
Printed in the USA
BVHW052234141119
563852BV00007B/126/P